Global Public Health:
A new era

Global Public Health: A new era

Edited by

Robert Beaglehole
University of Auckland, New Zealand

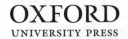

OXFORD
UNIVERSITY PRESS

Great Clarendon Street, Oxford OX2 6DP

Oxford University Press is a department of the University of Oxford. It
furthers the University's objective of excellence in research, scholarship,
and education by publishing worldwide in

Oxford New York

Auckland Bangkok Buenos Aires Cape Town Chennai
Dar es Salaam Delhi Hong Kong Istanbul Karachi Kolkata
Kuala Lumpur Madrid Melbourne Mexico City Mumbai
Nairobi São Paulo Shanghai Taipei Tokyo Toronto

Oxford is a registered trade mark of Oxford University Press in the UK
and in certain other countries

Published in the United States by Oxford University Press Inc., New York

A catalogue record for this title is avialable from the British Library

Library of Congress Cataloging in Publication Data

(Data available)

ISBN 0 19 851529 4 (Pbk)

10 9 8 7 6 5 4 3 2 1

Typeset by Newgen Imaging Systems (P) Ltd, Chennai, India
Printed in Great Britain
on acid-free paper by
Biddles Ltd., Guildford and King's Lynn

Editor's dedication
To Ruth Bonita and the next generation of the global public
health workforce

Preface

The aim of *Global public health: A new era* is to promote the practice of public health in all countries, with an emphasis on developing countries. It stems from the evidence that public health as a discipline and set of activities has for too long been neglected. The reinvigoration of public health practice is long overdue; it is time for public health practitioners to prepare for the long delayed "golden age." This reinvigoration needs to be based on a realistic assessment of the challenges to be faced and the current state of public health practice globally. This is the justification for this book.

Public health is the organized global and local effort to promote and protect the health of populations and to reduce health inequalities. The scope of public health practice is broad and ranges from the control of communicable diseases to the leadership of intersectoral efforts to improve health. The key public health perspective is the population-wide approach to the prevention and control of health problems.

The public health workforce includes people who are involved in protecting and promoting the collective health of whole or specific populations (as distinct from activities directed to patient care). The public health workforce is characterised by its diversity and its complexity and includes people from a wide range of occupational backgrounds. An effective public health workforce is central to the improvement of health system performance in all countries; it contributes to the organization, delivery, and evaluation of health services directed towards both individuals and populations and leads efforts to ensure the health enhancing effects of other related sectors.

Despite impressive health gains in almost all countries over the last few decades, the challenges facing the public health workforce are great and even more difficult to address than in the past. The unfinished agenda of communicable disease control is now greatly complicated by the emergence of new pandemics, notably HIV/AIDS and noncommunicable diseases, the effects of violence in all its manifestations, and global health threats, such as environmental changes. The events of 11 September 2001 in New York, the anthrax attacks in the USA and the subsequent "war on terrorism" have further widened the scope of public health.

Global public health: A new era grew out of a series of papers published in The Lancet in August and September 2000. The overarching theme of the series was the current state of public health theory and practice in the new and changing global context. The general theme of *Global public health* is similar to that of The Lancet series. Specifically, *Global public health* addresses three major issues: the changing global context for public health; the state of public health theory and practice in developed and developing countries; and strategies for strengthening the practice of public health in the twenty-first century.

This book is in three parts. The first part has two aims. Firstly, it surveys the complex old and new challenges facing public health practitioners. Secondly, it summarises the state of health globally using new data based on measures developed by the Word Health Organization and other groups to better describe population health status and trends.

Part two presents the first detailed review of the global state of public health. It analyses the public health situation in all regions of the world. Six chapters cover Europe, North and Latin America, and Australia and New Zealand. Three chapters cover China, Sub-Saharan Africa, and South Asia. The lessons from these chapters are surprisingly similar: the challenges are great; the public health workforce and infrastructure have long been neglected; and much needs to be done to reinvigorate the practice of public health.

The third section covers several cross cutting themes: the impact of the new public health threat from bioterrorism and its implications for the future of public health practice; the developing field of international public health ethics; and the central and neglected role of the public in strengthening the practice of public health. The final chapter summarises the major themes of the book and explores the opportunities for building the capacity of the public health workforce to respond to the major global health needs. Despite the enormity of the challenges facing public health practitioners, especially in developing countries, the tone adopted in the final section of this book is relatively optimistic. Perhaps this is a defensive reaction, but it is hard to imagine the global health situation improving, especially for the most disadvantaged populations, whether in poor or wealthy countries, without the efforts of a strong public health workforce.

This book is not a manual of public health practice; excellent handbooks already exist [1]. Nor is at an encyclopaedia of public health methods and issues; again the details can be found elsewhere [2].

The prime audience for *Global public health* is public health practition-ers and public health students in developed and developing countries. After all, if this audience is not more fully engaged with the issues dis-cussed in this book, the prospects for health of all populations will be bleaker than they should be. The book will also be of interest to a more general audience with a concern for global health issues.

It has been a pleasure editing this book and I pay tribute to all the contributors.

References

[1] Penchen D, Guest C, Melzer D, Muir Gray JA (eds.). *Oxford Handbook of Public Health Practice*. Oxford: Oxford University Press, 2001.

[2] Detels R, McEwen J, Beaglehole R, Tanaka H (eds.). *Oxford Textbook of Public Health*, 4th edn. Oxford: Oxford University Press, 2002.

Robert Beaglehole   November 2002

Contents

Contributors

Robert Beaglehole trained in medicine in New Zealand and in epidemiology and public health at the London School of Hygiene and Tropical Medicine and the University of North Carolina at Chapel Hill. He is on leave from his position as Professor of Community Health at the University of Auckland, New Zealand and working as a public health adviser in the Department of Health Service Provision at the World Health Organization, Geneva on strengthening the public health workforce in developing countries. He has published over 200 scientific papers, several books co-authored with Ruth Bonita on epidemiology and public health, and is co-editor of the Oxford Textbook of Public Health, Fourth Edition.

Ruth Bonita is Director of Surveillance, Noncommunicable Disease and Mental Health, at the World Health Organization, Geneva. She is responsible for mapping the advancing epidemics of NCDs and the major risk factors which predict them. The surveillance activities are focused on mid and low income countries where the gaps in information for policy are the greatest. Dr Bonita adopts a broad public health perspective to her work and is the author of many publications and scientific reports. She is co-author with Robert Beaglehole of a number of books on epidemiology and public health.

Richard A. Cash a Senior Lecturer and the Director of the Program on Ethical Issues in International Health Research in the Department of International Health at the Harvard School of Public Health. The program has recently conducted a number of workshops on research ethics in Latin America, Africa, the Middle East and Asia. He began international health work at what is now the International Centre for Diarrheal Disease Research and conducted the first clinical and field studies of Oral Rehydration Therapy. The epidemiology of new and reemerging infections and the impact of these on the development of societies is another research interest.

Peter Davis is Professor of Public Health at the Christchurch School of Medicine and Health Science, University of Otago, New Zealand. He is a social scientist and trained in sociology and in statistics from the London School of Economics, and in public health at the University of Auckland. Health services and health policy research have been a consistent theme of his work, most recently in the quality of care. He has published about a dozen books and over a hundred articles, and was recently appointed a Senior Editor with the international journal *Social Science and Medicine*.

Delanyo Dovlo qualified as a physician in Ghana and later studied Public Health and Human Resources in Leeds (UK) and Emory (USA) Universities respectively. He was Director of Human Resources in Ministry of Health in Ghana and prior to this spent several years as a District Medical Officer in rural health services. He also qualified as Member of the West African College of Physicians (Community Health). Outside Ghana, he has had experience as a consultant in District Health Systems and Human Resources Development in several African countries. He is currently the advisor on DFID's Management Strengthening Project in Namibia.

Sian Griffiths is Senior Fellow in Public Health at Oxford University and Visiting Professor at Brookes University. Until recently she was also Director of Public Health and Health Policy for the Oxfordshire Health Authority. She has authored and edited a variety of health-related publications. Between 1995 and 1999 she was Co-Chair of the Association for Public Health and Treasurer of the Faculty of Public Health Medicine. She is now President of the Faculty, a Board Member of the New Opportunities Fund, and a member of the National Cancer Taskforce.

Richard Horton trained in medicine in England. He joined The Lancet in 1990, opened the New York editorial office of the journal in 1993, and became Editor-in-Chief in 1995. He is a visiting professor at the London School of Hygiene and Tropical Medicine, a past president of the World Association of Medical Editors, and a fellow of the UK's Academy of Medical Sciences. He has a particular editorial interest in health and development issues.

T Jacob John trained in medicine, pediatrics and infectious diseases and in virology in India, the UK and USA. After serving the Christian Medical College, Vellore, India for over 30 years as Pediatrician and Virologist, he retired from service and is currently Advisor to the Ministry of Health in Kerala State, establishing district level disease surveillance and a Public Health Institute of Virology and Infectious Diseases. He has published over 300 scientific papers. In 1994 he was the President of the Indian

Association of Medical Microbiologists and in 1999 the President of the Indian Academy of Pediatrics.

Henri Jouval Jr trained in medicine and internal medicine in Brazil. He is currently Country Representative of the Pan-American Health Organization in Mexico. He has worked as PAHO Country Representative in Argentina. He was Secretary of Medical Care of the National Directorate of the former National Institute of Medical Care of the Social Security and Secretary of Planning and Budgeting of National Directorate of the former National Institute of Medical Care of the Social Security. He was Associate Professor of the Faculty of Medicine of the Federal University of Rio de Janeiro. He has published over 90 papers on public health.

John Last, a graduate of the University of Adelaide medical school, is emeritus professor of epidemiology at the University of Ottawa. He trained in epidemiology at the MRC Social Medicine Research Unit, London, England, and has worked in many countries. He is the editor of the *Dictionary of Epidemiology*, former editor-in-chief of *Public Health and Preventive Medicine* ("Maxcy-Rosenau-Last"); author or editor of several other books and medical journals, chapters in forty five books and over 200 original articles. His awards include MD honoris causa,Uppsala University; the Duncan Clark Award (for contributions to preventive medicine); and the Abraham Lilienfeld Award (for contributions to epidemiology).

Liming Lee graduated from Beijing Medical University in 1982 and received the MPH degree at department of epidemiology in the same university in 1986. He was a visiting professor at School of Public Health, Hawaii University from 1987–88. As a post-doctoral fellow, he worked at Johns Hopkins University from 1990–91. From 1995 he has been Dean of the School of Public Health, Beijing Medical University and is Assistant President of Peking University and Vice President of Peking University Health Science Center. He is now Director of Chinese Center for Disease Control and Prevention. He is deputy chief-editor of Chinese Journal of Public Health and Chinese Journal of Non-communicable Disease Prevention and Control.

Uta Lehmann has a background in social sciences and worked in health personnel education for the past eleven years. She is particularly involved in the area of human resource development for health through teaching course development, research and publications. She is a member of the academic staff at the University of the Western Cape, Cape Town.

Vivian Lin is the Professor of Public Health and Head of School at La Trobe University, in Melbourne, Australia and was previously the Executive Officer for the Australian National Public Health Partnership. She trained in political science and biology at Yale University and public health at UC Berkeley and has worked in governments and universities in the US as well as Australia. She has had long associations with health policy in China, as a consultant for the World Bank, World Health Organisation, and AusAID.

Sarah Macfarlane is an Associate Director in the Health Equity Theme of the Rockefeller Foundation, and previously a Reader in Statistics and Epidemiology in the Liverpool School of Tropical Medicine at the University of Liverpool, UK. She has collaborated in a large number of research and training projects in sub-Saharan Africa and South East Asia, and has published widely. Her quantitative background, combined with a conviction that equity in health can only be achieved through a process that is itself equitable, has led her to search for a balance between quantitative and qualitative approaches to public health.

Cristiani Vieira Machado trained in medicine and is currently a doctoral student in public health planning in Brazil. She also trained as a specialist in Governmental Management at the Brazilian National School of Public Administration. She has worked as a public health officer at the federal, state and municipal levels and participated in research projects on public health. She currently works at the Brazilian Ministry of Health, in the Department of Health System Decentralization, where she coordinates activities of support to states and municipalities.

Martin McKee trained in medicine in Northern Ireland and in public health at the London School of Hygiene and Tropical Medicine where he is now Professor of European Public Health and co-director of the school's European Centre on Health of Societies in Transition and one of the Research Directors of the European Observatory on Health Care Systems (www.observatory.dk). His research is focused on health and health policy in central and eastern Europe and the former Soviet Union. He has published over 250 scientific papers, is editor or author of nine books, and editor in chief of the European Journal of Public Health.

Tony McMichael is Director, National Centre for Epidemiology and Population Health, Australian National University, Canberra. Previously he was Professor of Epidemiology at the London School of Hygiene and Tropical Medicine. His research has encompassed occupational diseases, diet and cancer, and environmental health hazards. He has a major interest in assessing the health risks from global environmental change, having contributed to the UN's Intergovernmental Panel on Climate Change. He is a member of the International Science Panel on Population and Environment. He has published several books on global environmental health issues.

Colin Mathers trained in theoretical physics in Australia but has spent much of his career developing population health monitoring systems for Australia at the Australian Institute of Health and Welfare. He joined the Global Program on Evidence for Health Policy at the World Health Organization, Geneva in 2000 and has played a leading role in the Global Burden of Disease 2000 project and in the development of summary measures of population health. He has published over sixty scientific papers, several books on population health and burden of disease, and is a co-editor of the journal Population Health Metrics.

Wilma Meeus studied medicine in the Netherlands and is enrolled in the MPH programme of the School of Public Health at the University of the Western Cape, Cape Town. Since 1985, she has been involved in addressing public health issues in complex emergencies, mainly on the African continent (Sudan, Somalia, Uganda, Zaire and Rwanda) as well as in Kosovo and India. This involvement has ranged from advising national/local Ministries of Health on policy development and planning, and on the establishment of multidisciplinary Disaster Management structures to providing advice and assistance in establishing (post-conflict) NGO coordination procedures.

José Noronha trained in medicine, public health and social medicine in Brazil and England. He is Associate Professor of the Department of Health Policy, Planning and Administration of the Institute of Social Medicine of the State University of Rio de Janeiro, and researcher of the Department of Health Information of the Oswaldo Cruz Foundation, Rio de Janeiro. He is currently President of the Brazilian Association of Public Health (Associação Brasileira de Saúde Coletiva—ABRASCO), Councilor of the National Health Council, Ministry of Health of Brazil, where he coordinates the Commission of Science and Technology in Health. He has been State Secretary of Health of Rio de Janeiro, Brazil.

Gudrun Persson has a Master of Business Administration from Gothenburg School of Economics and studied epidemiology and public health at the Karolinska Institute in Stockholm. She works as a senior researcher at the Centre for Epidemiology at The National Board of Health and Welfare. She is the project leader of the Swedish National Public Health Report.

John Raeburn trained in psychology, and holds various positions in the Faculty of Medical and Health Sciences in the University of Auckland, New Zealand. These include Director of Health Promotion, Director of Mental Health Programmes, Director of the Community Office, Assistant Dean, Health Science and Public Health, and Associate Professor of Behavioural Science. He has had thirty years experience working in the areas of health promotion, mental health and community development, has authored more than 60 academic papers in these areas, and is author with Irving Rootman of People-Centred Health Promotion.

David Sanders trained in medicine in Zimbabwe and in paediatrics and public health in Britain. Between 1981 and 1992 he was a member of the academic staff of University of Zimbabwe Medical School. In 1993 he became founding Director and Professor of the School of Public Health at the University of the Western Cape which provides practice-oriented postgraduate and continuing education and undertakes research in public health and primary health care. He has been actively involved in the health policy process in both Zimbabwe and South Africa, particularly in the areas of nutrition and human resource development. He is author of two books on health, development and primary health care.

F. Douglas Scutchfield is the Peter P Bosomworth Professor of Health Services Research and Policy at the University of Kentucky. He holds academic appointments in the College of Medicine, College of Allied Health and Martin School of Public Policy and Administration. He is Director of the Kentucky School of Public Health, Associate Dean of the College of Medicine, Director of the Center for Health Services Management and Research, and Chair of the Department of Health Services. He trained in medicine at the University of Kentucky and is a Fellow of the American College of Preventive Medicine and the American Academy of Family Physicians.

Stig Wall has been professor of Epidemiology and Health Care Research, Umeå International School of Public Health, Sweden, since 1986. His training is in social sciences. He has served on several national and international funding and health policy agencies to assess and initiate research and health interventions. He is scientific adviser to the Swedish National Board of Health and Social Welfare and Board member of its Epidemiological Centre. He chairs the peer review board of health research at Sida/SAREC and has chaired the Swedish Epidemiological Association. He is currently chief editor of the *Scandinavian Journal of Public Health*.

Ruotao Wang is the Professor of Epidemiology and Public Health in Union School of Public Health, Beijing. He graduated from Tianjin

Medical University, China, in 1968 with a major in Medicine. He trained in epidemiology at the London School of Hygiene and Tropical Medicine and in law at the Yale Law School. He has taught epidemiology, biostatistics and other courses in public health, and conducted research and field studies in China. He is currently working in the research of public health law and information resources development in National Center for AIDS Control & Prevention, China.

Lars Weinehall is a specialist in family medicine and received his PhD in epidemiology in 1997. Since 1985 he has coordinated the Västerbotten Intervention Programme. His main research interest is cardiovascular disease prevention, especially the role of primary health care providers. He is a member of the Swedish Physicians Association Task Force on Prevention, the Parliamentary Commission on Health Statistics, the National Public Health Commission and the Parliamentary Commission on Research Ethics.

Franklin White is Professor and Chair, Community Health Sciences, The Aga Khan University, Pakistan and honorary Adjunct Professor, Dalhousie University, Canada. He initiated the Canadian Field Epidemiology program (1976), is Past President, Canadian Public Health Association (1986–88), and formerly a Director, Canadian Society for International Health. He was with the World Health Organization Regional Office for the Americas (PAHO/WHO) and served as Director, Caribbean Epidemiology Center (1989–95), and initiated the Regional Program on Non-Communicable Diseases (1995–98). He received the PAHO/WHO Medal of Honor (1997). He has published over 250 scientific papers. Based in Pakistan since 1998, he has also served as a public health consultant elsewhere in Asia.

Daniel Wikler is Professor of Ethics and Population Health at the Harvard School of Public Health. He served as President of the International Association of Bioethics and the American Association of Bioethics, and was Senior Staff Ethicist at the World Health Organization from 1999 to 2001, where he was concerned with resource allocation, experimentation with human subjects, and other ethical issues in global public health. His *From Chance to Choice: Genetics and Justice*, co-authored with three fellow philosophers, was published by Cambridge University Press in 2000.

Witold Zatonski is Director, Division of Epidemiology and Cancer Prevention at the Maria Sklodowska-Curie Memorial Cancer Centre in Warsaw. His department is a World Health Organization Collaborating Center for the Action Plan for Tobacco Free Europe. His work concentrates on defining causes of premature death and intervention activities to reduce morbidity and mortality, particularly from cancer, in Poland and Eastern Europe. He has authored over 300 publications. He is a member of the Committee of Epidemiology and Public Health at the Polish Academy of Science whose national and international contribution to health has been recognized by many prestigious awards.

Hongwen Zhao is enrolled in a DrPH at La Trobe Uiversity, Melbourne. He trained in medicine and public health in China and the USA. He has been a project manager in the Foreign Loan Office of the Ministry of Health, China and a health specialist in the World Bank Beijing Office.

Chapter 1

The global context for public health

Tony McMichael and Robert Beaglehole

Introduction

A major transition in the health of human populations is underway. In most populations there have been impressive gains in life expectancy during the past half-century. Fertility rates have been generally declining over the past several decades. The profile of major causes of death and disease is being transformed; in developing countries, noncommunicable diseases are replacing the long-dominant infectious diseases. Meanwhile, the pattern of infectious diseases, internationally, has become much more labile, and antimicrobial resistance is increasing.

The prospects for population health depend to an increasing, but still uncertain, extent on the varied effects of globalization. This is particularly so in the world's less wealthy populations. This topic is contentious, and hampered by a lack of systematic research evidence [1,2]. Health prospects also depend on trends in global environmental conditions, occurring in response to the pressures of economic activity. These relationships are at the heart of the nascent "sustainability transition" debate [3]. Overall, public health is at a substantive crossroads [4].

Improvements in the health status of western populations during the past two centuries have resulted primarily from broad-based changes in the social, dietary and material environments, shaped in part by improved sanitation and other deliberate public health interventions [5]. In less-developed countries, more recently health gains have occurred in the wake of increased literacy, family spacing, improved nutrition and vector control, assisted by the transfer of knowledge about sanitation, vaccination and treatment of infectious diseases [6].

This history of the fundamental influence on population health of social, economic and technological changes is a reminder to public health researchers and practitioners, and those in the political and public realms with whom they interact, that they should take a broad view of the determinants of population health. This requires an ecological view of health. That is, it requires an awareness that shifts in the ecology of human living in relation to both the natural and social environments account for much of the ebb and flow of diseases over time [7].

In this chapter we describe this larger-scale context within which public health researchers and practitioners should address both traditional and new challenges to population health. These challenges are heightened by the even more fundamental, and unfamiliar, challenge of ensuring the sustainability of humankind's social and economic activities.

The scope of public health

Broadly defined, public health is the art and science of preventing disease, promoting population health, and extending life through organized local and global efforts [8]. Two aspects of this public health task have been claiming increasing attention. First, because social and material inequalities within a society generate health inequalities, a central task is to identify, through research, the underlying political, social and behavioral determinants of these health inequalities [9]. That knowledge must then be applied, in part through professional practice, to the development and implementation of effective social policies. In its fullest sense, this must include the lessening of social inequalities. Second, longer-term changes in the structure and conditions of both the social and natural environments will affect the sustainability of good health within populations. A ready example is the rapid rise of obesity in urban populations everywhere, as ways-of-living become less physically active. Public health, as Virchow pointed out more than a century ago, is "politics writ large".

The goals of contemporary public health effort must encompass these larger-scale dimensions: the improvement of population health; the reduction of social and health inequalities; and the striving for health-sustaining environments. In traditional, largely self-contained, agrarian-based societies that produce, consume and trade on a local basis and with low-impact technologies, the social and environmental determinants of health are predominantly local and relatively circumscribed. However, the industrialization and modernization over the past century have altered the scale of contact, influence and exchange between societies. Further, it has institutionalized hierarchical economic relations, reinforcing the modern world's "structured unfairness,"[10] and has exacerbated the rich-poor gap worldwide and increased the scale of human impact on the environment [11].

An important step towards addressing the goals of public health has been the recent affirmation that a population's health reflects more than the simple summation of the risk-factor profile and health status of its individual members. It is also a collective characteristic that reflects the population's social history and its cultural, material, and ecological circumstances [12–14]. Epidemiological analysis confined to studying "risk factor" differences between individuals gives little insight into variations in population health indices, either between populations or in any particular population over time. For example, the effect of heatwaves and cold spells on mortality differs between European populations at low and high latitudes, reflecting differences in culture, housing design, and environmental conditioning [15]. The inverse relationship seen in more-developed countries between the within-population income gradient and average life expectancy [16] cannot be satisfactorily explained at the individual level, even though mediating biomedical pathways that relate to individual experiences of stress, status or deprivation may be identified. Likewise, the apparent surge in excessive alcohol consumption that occurred in post-communist Russia [17] is essentially a population-level process that can only partly be understood by elucidating concomitant individual-level phenomena. The individual-level perspective fails to conceptualise the population's health both as something that reflects prevailing ecological conditions and as a public good that affects social functioning, community morale, and collective economic performance [18]. Thus, analyses at the individual, community and whole-population levels can address complementary, qualitatively distinct, types of questions [7].

The public health endeavor is thus a broad and inclusive enterprise that extends to political, social, and environmental leadership and management. Clinical medicine is part of this overall public health effort to promote and protect population health, and to reduce the impact of illness and disease. In a rapidly changing world, with new and larger-scale influences on population health, implementing a broad-based, multi-sectored, public health effort becomes an increasingly important challenge. Currently, there is little evidence that the public health workforce is equipped to meet these challenges.

Health and sustainable development

The term "sustainable development" has great elasticity. In its crudest form, it is used to refer to achieving an economic system that can continue to grow, at least over the foreseeable future. Recent insights have extended the concept by embedding the human-made economic system within the wider biosphere: "sustainability" thus means that economic development must occur within the constraints of maintaining intact the ecosystems that support human societies and the things that they value [19].

Human population health is widely viewed as an incidental beneficiary of the process of development, which has as its central goal economic growth. In some formulations [20] population health has been viewed primarily from a utilitarian perspective, as an *input* to economic development. The healthier the population, the more efficient its economic functioning: health thus facilitates the acquisition of wealth. This perspective is also evident in the recent work of World Health Organization's (WHO) Commission on Macroeconomics and Health which, while recognizing the importance of health in its own right, emphasizes the potential contribution of investing in health to promote economic growth [21]. The danger is that this formulation treats economic growth as the primary desired endpoint and neglects the broader consequences of this growth, including its medium-to-longer-term impacts on environment and health.

The mainstream perspective on economic development has not yet incorporated the notion that "health" is an *ecological* characteristic of populations, reflecting the wider conditions of the social and natural environments. Rather, "health" is considered primarily at the personal and family level. In developed countries, health has become largely commodified as an asset to be managed by personal behavioral choices and personal access to the formal health care system. This perspective ignores the ecological dimension, where the health of a population also reflects the level of biological (including mental) functioning that is permitted by the environment.

In animal and plant populations, the size of the population and its "health" reflects the carrying capacity of the environment for that species. That is, the environment determines the maximum number that can be supported, and that number is the "carrying capacity" of the local habitat [7]. In contrast, human populations are not exclusively constrained by the prevailing environmental conditions; humans, through culture and technology, can increase the carrying capacity of their local environments—at least temporarily. In the longer term, the sustainability of this amplified carrying capacity becomes an issue. The sustained good health of any population requires a stable and productive natural environment that: yields assured supplies of food and fresh water; has a relatively constant climate in which climate-sensitive physical and biological systems do not change for the worse; and retains biodiversity (a fundamental source of both present and future value). For the human species the stability, richness and equity of the social environment (i.e., "social capital") are also important to population health [22].

Population health is, therefore, more than just a utilitarian input or an incidental consequence of economic development. It should be a *central focus of development*. The purpose of societal "development" and, specifically of public health activity, is to improve the conditions, enjoyment and healthiness of life for human societies and to do so in a way that entails sharing those benefits equitably. If the development process is not conducive to sustained and equitable improvements in health, then in a very fundamental sense it is not "sustainable development".

Human ecology as a determinant of population health

Changes in human culture over many centuries have resulted in major shifts in the patterns of population health [3]. A central example, ongoing over the past 10,000 years since human societies first began farming, has been the nutritional impact of traditional staple-based, often monotonous, agrarian diets. Prior to the "second agricultural revolution" beginning in Europe in the nineteenth century, most agrarian societies had widespread malnutrition and recurring famines [23]. The geographic spread of human populations has compounded this nutritional deficiency problem. For example, the extension of agrarian societies into highland regions and arid regions exposed many populations to dietary iodine deficiency, leading to iodine deficiency disorders [24]. Nevertheless, because of the great increase in environmental carrying capacity conferred by agricultural production and trade, farming populations have generally outnumbered and replaced smaller hunter-gatherer populations.

Many of the diseases that characterize modern wealthy societies, and increasingly poor societies, reflect a discordance between evolved biological needs and contemporary ways of living [25,26]. For example, the radical industrial transformation of the food supply, entailing huge shifts in levels of consumption of saturated fats, simple sugars, salt and dietary fibre, contributed to the noncommunicable disease epidemics (cardiovascular disease, diabetes, various cancers) that characterize longer-living populations in developed countries and, increasingly, developing countries [27]. Urban crowding and migration have facilitated the local and long-distance spread of infectious diseases, respectively. Physical inactivity in the modern, mechanized, increasingly urban environment predisposes to the worldwide rising prevalence of obesity.

Nevertheless, various social and technical advances over the past two centuries have brought marked reductions in mortality, particularly in early life, with resultant gains in life expectancy, and an ensuing reduction in birth rates. This composite process, the demographic transition, continues to transform life expectancies and patterns of disease in developing countries.

Explanations for recent trends in population health

There have been broad gains in life expectancy over the past half-century, and these gains are continuing in most regions [3,28]. Setbacks have occurred, however, in sub-Saharan Africa, primarily because of the ravages of HIV/AIDS, and in some of the former socialist countries of Central and Eastern Europe because of the turbulent social and economic disruptions that occurred in the early 1990s. Fertility rates are now declining on a wide front, and there have been widespread gains in maternal mortality and infant and child survival in developing countries. World population is, on current projections, expected to flatten out at around 8–9 billion by 2050, gaining up to another one billion by 2100—a lesser figure than previously predicted.

The profile of major causes of death and disease is being transformed. As traditional infectious diseases continue to recede in many poorer countries, the incidence of chronic noncommunicable diseases of mid and later adulthood is rising in all developing countries. Meanwhile, there is concern over the increasingly labile pattern of "emerging and resurging" infectious diseases [29]. More generally, health inequalities between rich and poor nations and rich and poor population subgroups persist.

It was long assumed that the decline in fatal infection in industrializing western societies was largely attributable to their "conquest" by effective specific counter-measures, most recently by vaccines and antibiotics and earlie by sanitation and improved water supplies. However, Thomas McKeown, using historical English data, showed that vaccines and antibiotics came too late to make major contributions [30]. Over 90 percent of the recorded decline in tuberculosis mortality in England, for example, occurred before the advent of chemotherapy in the late 1940s. McKeown argued that improved nutrition, by enhancing host resistance, was the main determinant of the modern decline in fatal infection. The substantial historical increase in body size in wealthy countries attests to improved nutrition in infancy and childhood. The relationship between child nutrition and infection is generally reciprocal: better nourished children are more resistant to death from infection and protection against infection reduces the nutrient losses caused by infection.

However, it is too simple to suppose that the benefits of new knowledge flow exclusively from their application by clinical and public health professionals. How parents care for their children appears to be crucially important because the chances of children surviving are improved when their parents have been to school. This effect of parental education is very powerful when compared to other potential determinants of child mortality in low and middle-income countries. Thus "medicine" and "public health" need to be interpreted in explanatory models as possessions of a whole society— individuals, families, communities and larger social formations— and not just as domains of professional practice [31].

India illustrates how mortality can decline in a low-income country even though improvements in the conditions of living have been relatively slow [32]. Mortality in India declined markedly through the twentieth century from very high levels that prevailed around 1900. By the mid-1990s, the chance of dying before age fifteen had been reduced by about three quarters to around 13 percent and the chance of dying between ages fifteen and sixty-five had been reduced by about two-thirds, to under 30 percent. Within India, mortality decline has been much more strongly associated, geographically, with institutional modernization (as indicated by high school attendance rates for girls in rural areas) than with rising incomes.

The mortality decline in the second half of the twentieth century was even more rapid in East Asia (notwithstanding China's catastrophic famine in 1959–61) and in Latin America. For adult males, mortality levels in Chinese cities are now amongst the most favorable in the world, as are those in Caribbean states such as Jamaica and Cuba. Mortality decline has been much slower in sub-Saharan Africa. In some countries severely effected by HIV (such as Zimbabwe and Zambia) and by civil war (such as Rwanda and Liberia), life expectancy fell in the last two decades of the twentieth century.

The most persuasive explanations of mortality decline in low- and middle-income countries involve improvements in three domains: improvements in the material conditions of life (indicated, for example, by real incomes or child growth rates); institutional change, especially schooling for girls; and increases in knowledge and in its application. The reductions in mortality at any particular population income level are mainly attributable to increases in the stock of scientific and practical knowledge and institutional changes that help to put this knowledge to work, especially schooling for girls. One attempt to attribute credit for increased life expectancy in

115 low- and middle-income countries between 1960 and 1990, allocated 20 percent to increased real incomes and 30 percent to schooling for girls; the residual 50 percent being allocated to the generation and use of new knowledge [18].

Each of these three "factors" is serving as a marker for wider and more complex social and economic processes. Thus economic development brings not only increases in private incomes but also increases in capital stocks, many of a public nature: roads and schools are built; teachers are trained; electronic communications are improved. Changes in these economic "stocks" could be at least as important for health protection as increases in economic "flows" (income). A marked degree of female autonomy is probably central to exceptional mortality declines, especially in poor but open societies. When there is no scandal about girls assuming roles outside the house even when they are unmarried but have reached puberty, or about older women appearing in public on their own initiative, then girls are more likely to remain at school, and mothers are more likely to take action about sick children or about themselves, and, when necessary will travel to health centres, wait in queues of mixed sex, and argue with male physicians [33].

The increases in knowledge that have contributed to mortality decline are also likely to be complex. For example, approximately 80 percent of the world's children were estimated to have been immunised against measles in 1997, up from about 50 percent in 1987. The knowledge contributing to this protection against early death extends from the scientific knowledge embedded in the vaccine, to the technical knowledge embedded in the "cold chains" used to convey vaccines safely to remote areas, and also to the "organizational knowledge" about the best way of conducting immunization programmes. And new knowledge embedded in communications technologies almost certainly helped in the planning, promotion and conduct of these programmes.

Globalization: Setting the scene

"Globalization" like "sustainable development", is an elastic term. Here we use it to refer to the increasing interconnectedness of countries through cross-border flows of goods, services, money, people, information and ideas; the increasing openness of countries to such flows; and the development of international rules and institutions dealing with cross-border flows. This is not a new phenomenon, although the current phase of globalization, dating from the 1980s, has seen an exceptionally rapid increase in interconnectedness and by more radical changes in the international institutional framework than previous phases [34]. The core component of globalization is economic interconnectedness, including the associated ascendancy of deregulated markets in international trade and investment. Two other important domains are technological globalization, especially of information and communication technologies, and cultural globalization where popular culture is increasingly dominated by the United States and the English language. There is also an emerging globalization of ethical and judicial standards which may render social and individual rights more secure (see Chapter 13).

Economic "globalization" has been a long-evolving feature of a world dominated by western society. The onset of the twentieth century was a time of vigoros free trade, subsequently curtailed in the aftermath of World War I. Contemporary globalization differs in both the scale and the comprehensiveness of change, and in the associated decline in the country's capacity to set social policy [35,36]. The Western world's post-World War I international development project initially anticipated that countries everywhere would converge towards the Western model of national democratic capitalism. However, this project has evolved towards the building of an integrated and deregulated free-market global economy. These globalizing processes, in turn, have become a major determinant of national, social, and economic policies [37,38]. Thus, although responsibility for healthcare and the public health system remains with national governments, the fundamental social, economic, and environmental determinants of population health are increasingly supranational. This combination of liberal economic structures and domestic policy constraint promotes socioeconomic inequalities and political instability, each of which adversely affects population health. Unless the moderating role of the state or of international agencies is strengthened, increasing competition for the world's limited natural resources is likely to damage intercountry relations, local and global environments, and population health [37].

The principal promoters of a globalized market-based economic system are international agencies such as the World Bank, the International Monetary Fund (IMF), and transnational corporations. The main strategies have included the promotion of free trade through the rules of the World Trade Organisation (WTO) and its Multilateral Trade Agreements (MTAs), corporate taxation concessions and investment incentives allied to relaxation of wage controls and workplace standards, and the contraction of national public-sector spending in the health, education, and welfare sectors.

Structural adjustment programmes imposed by the IMF on the economies of many poor countries, promoting particularly the wealth-creating role of the private sector, have often impaired population health. The curtailment of education under this imposed regime of economic rationalism has threatened advances in literacy in women, fertility reduction, and improved reproductive health [39]. The World Bank now recognizes the need for a strong State to carry out essential public functions, including public health, and to ensure well-functioning markets [40]. Meanwhile, tension persists between the philosophy of neoliberalism, emphasizing the self-interest of market-based economics, and the philosophy of social justice that sees collective responsibility and benefit as the prime social goal. The practice of public health, with its underlying community and population perspective, sits more comfortably with the latter philosophy.

The mainstream economic view is that opening the world's economy increases trade which in turn increases growth, especially in poorer countries [1]. National economic growth then increases incomes, especially for the poor, and increasing income provides more resources for health services at the same time as increasing the incomes of the poor improves their health. In brief, opening the economy improves health [41]. If the mainstream economic view were correct, then one would expect to see the increasing openness of economies over recent decades contributing to an acceleration in economic growth. In fact, the growth rate of the world economy has slowed down dramatically as the pace of economic opening has accelerated—it was nearly halved from 3.4 percent in the 1960s to 1.8 percent in the 1970s, and more than halved again to 0.8 percent in 1990–98 [2]. Of course, many other factors must be considered before this could be considered as clear evidence that opening a national economy can slow economic growth, but it does raise serious questions about the most basic tenet of the prevailing economic view. Such doubts are reinforced by systematic methodological flaws in cross-country studies purporting to provide evidence for linkage from openness to growth [42].

As economic liberalization has accelerated, there has also been a polarization between richer and poorer countries [2]. Again, this is the opposite of what mainstream economics predicts. Over the long term, few developing countries have experienced a decline in the proportion of their population living in poverty. Most countries for which data are available, representing nearly half the world's population, have experienced increasing inequality, while the remainder either show no clear trend or do not have sufficient data to make an assessment. There is some indication that the trend has become less favorable: 44 percent of the world population live in countries where inequality first declined then increased, while only

1 percent live in countries where the opposite occurred (again, based on countries with adequate data) [2].

Income disparity has increased between high- and low-income countries and within many countries. Both trends have contributed to an increase in overall global inequality. There have been increases in inequality in Asia and Africa, and a massive increase in Eastern Europe, with smaller declines in the developed countries and Latin America [43]. With a combination of slowing growth and increasing inequality at the global level, it is not surprising that progress in reducing poverty has been disappointing.

Alongside this economic globalization has been the rapid development and international spread of information and communication technologies, facilitated by investments in infrastructure, improved technologies, and shrinking costs. However, the reach of the telephone and internet is still limited within poor populations. Globally co-ordinated advertising, technological innovation, and marketing opportunities are increasingly driving modern consumer behaviors, as exemplified by the intensified global promotion of tobacco products [44].

Another feature of today's world is the increase in human mobility. Most movement is voluntary; some is involuntary and in response to conflict, civil disorder, and natural disaster. The number of environmental and political refugees has increased greatly over the past two decades, surging particularly in the late 1990s [45]. Increased mobility of labor can be of mutual economic benefit—many less-developed economies welcome cheap overseas labor, and international remittances from these workers assist their home economies. Meanwhile, human mobility is also important in the enhanced transmission of ideas, values, and microbiological agents.

Globalization and public health

From a public health perspective, globalization is having mixed effects [28,35,36]. On the one hand accelerated economic growth and technological advances have enhanced health and life expectancy in many populations. At least in the short-to-medium term, these material advances allied to social modernization and various health-care and public health programmes yield gains in population health. On the other hand, aspects of globalization jeopardise population health via the erosion of social and environmental conditions, the global division of labor, the exacerbation of the rich–poor income gap between and within countries, and the accelerating spread of consumerism (Box 1.1) [28].

One aspect of the growth in international trade with particularly deleterious public health consequences has been the escalation in the sales

Box 1.1   Examples of health risks posed by globalization

The primary health risks, a result of globalization on social and natural environments, include:

- Perpetuation and exacerbation of income differentials, both within and among countries, thereby creating and maintaining the basic poverty-associated conditions for poor health.

- The fragmentation and weakening of labor markets as internationally mobile capital acquires greater relative power and jeopardise the health of workers by encouraging a lowering of occupational health and safety standards.

- The consequences of global environmental changes (includes changes in atmospheric composition, land degradation, depletion of biodiversity, spread of "invasive" species, and dispersal of persistent organic pollutants).

Other, more specific, examples of risks to health include:

- The spread of tobacco-caused diseases as the tobacco industry globalizes its markets.

- The diseases of dietary excesses as food production and food processing become intensified and as urban consumer preferences are shaped by globally promoted images and mass marketing.

- The diverse public health consequences of the proliferation of private car ownership, as car manufacturers extend their marketing.

- The widespread rise of obesity in urban populations.

- Expansion of the international drug trade.

- Infectious diseases spreading more easily because of increased world-wide travel.

- The apparent increasing prevalence of depression and mental-health disorders in ageing and fragmented urban populations.

of weapons and associated equipment, much of it facilitated by western governments. sub-Saharan Africa provides many tragic examples of these effects as does the continuing instability in the Middle-East. The nature of modern conflict is such that most casualties are civilians, with women and children being particularly vulnerable [46].

Global environmental change and health

Over the past two centuries, three great changes in the human condition have occurred: industrialization, urbanization, and, latterly, increased control over human fertility. The associated combination of receding infant-and-child mortality, followed by a downtrend in adult mortality, rapid population growth and economic intensification, has resulted in humans exerting enormous aggregate pressure on the natural environment.

A major manifestation of this increasing scale of the human enterprise is the advent of global environmental changes. While not directly caused by the globalization processes discussed above, global environmental change reflects the increasing magnitude of human numbers and the intensity of modern consumer-driven economies [47]. Humankind is now disrupting at a global level some of the biosphere's life-support systems [48], which provide environmental stabilization, replenishment, organic production, cleansing of water and air and recycling of nutrient elements. These environmental "services" were taken for granted in a less populated, lower-impact world. However, today humankind is changing the gaseous composition of the lower and middle atmospheres; there is a net loss of productive soils on all continents, depletion of most ocean fisheries and many of the great aquifers upon which irrigated agriculture depends; and an unprecedented rate of loss rate of whole species and many local populations [7]. An estimated one-third of the world's stocks of natural ecological resources have been lost since 1970 [49]. These changes to Earth's basic life-supporting processes pose long-term risks to human population health [50].

Global climate change

Climate scientists forecast that the continued accumulation of heat-trapping greenhouse gases in the troposphere will change global patterns of temperature, precipitation and climatic variability over the coming decades [51]. A rise of 1–3 °C over the coming half-century, greater at high than at low latitudes, would occur faster than any rise encountered by humankind since the inception of agriculture around ten thousand years ago. The UN's Intergovernmental Panel on Climate Change and various other national scientific panels have assessed the potential health consequences of climate change [52–54]. These risks to human health will arise from increased exposures to thermal extremes and from regionally variable increases in weather disasters. Other risks would arise from the disruption of complex ecological systems that determine the geography of vector-borne infections (such as malaria, dengue fever and leishmaniasis), and the range, seasonality and incidence of various food-borne and water-borne infections, the yields of agricultural crops, the range of plant and livestock pests and pathogens, the salination of coastal lands and freshwater supplies due to sea-level rise, and the climatically-related production of photochemical air pollutants, spores and pollens.

Public health scientists now face the task of estimating, via interdisciplinary collaborations, the future health impacts of these projected scenarios of climatic-environmental conditions. Mathematical models have recently been used, for example, to estimate how climatic changes would affect the potential geographic range of vector-borne infectious diseases [55].

Stratospheric ozone depletion

Depletion of stratospheric ozone by human-made gases such as chlorofluorocarbons has occurred over recent decades and is likely to peak around 2020. Ambient ground-level ultraviolet irradiation is estimated to have increased consequently by up to 10 percent at mid-to-high latitudes over the past two decades [56]. Scenario-based modeling, integrating the processes of emissions accrual, ozone destruction, UVR flux, and cancer induction, indicates that the European and US populations will experience a resultant 5–10 percent excess in skin cancer incidence during the middle decades of the coming century [57].

Biodiversity loss and invasive species

As human demand for space, materials and food increases, so populations and species of plants and animals are being rapidly extinguished. An important consequence for humans is the disruption of ecosystems that provide "nature's goods and services"[35]. Biodiversity loss also means the loss, before discovery, of many of nature's chemicals and genes, of the kind that have already conferred enormous medical and health benefits. Myers estimates that five-sixths of tropical vegetative nature's medicinal goods have yet to be recruited for human benefit [58].

Meanwhile, "invasive" species are spreading worldwide into new non-natural environments via intensified human food production, commerce and mobility. The resultant changes in regional species composition have myriad consequences for human health. For example, the spread of water hyacinth in eastern Africa's Lake Victoria, introduced from Brazil as a decorative plant, is now a breeding ground for the water snail that transmits schistosomiasis and for the proliferation of diarrhoeal disease organisms [59].

Impairment of food-producing ecosystems

Increasing pressures of agricultural and livestock production are stressing the world's arable lands and pastures. The twenty-first century begins with an estimated one-third of the world's previously productive land seriously damaged, by erosion, compaction, salination, waterlogging and chemicalization that destroys organic content [60,61]. Similar pressures on the world's ocean fisheries have left most of them severely depleted or stressed [62]. Almost certainly we must find an environmentally benign, safe and socially acceptable way of using genetic engineering to increase food yields, if we are to produce sufficient food for another three billion persons (with higher expectations) over the coming half-century.

Modeling studies, allowing for future trends in trade and economic development, have estimated that climate change would cause a slight downturn globally of around 2–4 percent in cereal grain yields (which represent two-thirds of world food energy). The estimated downturn in yield would be considerably greater in the food-insecure regions in South Asia, the Middle East, North Africa and Central America [63,64].

Other global environmental changes

Freshwater aquifers in all continents are being depleted of their ancient "fossil water" supplies. Agricultural and industrial demand, amplified by population growth, often greatly exceeds the rate of natural recharge. Water-related political and public health crises loom within decades.

Various semi-volatile organic chemicals (such as polychlorinated biphenyls) are now disseminated worldwide, via a sequential "distillation" process in the cells of the lower atmosphere, thereby transferring chemicals from their usual origins in low to mid-latitudes to high latitudes. Increasingly high levels are occurring in polar mammals and fish and in the humans that eat them. Various chlorinated organic chemicals, butyltin and other compounds adversely affect the immune and reproductive systems of mammals, including humans. That is, chemical pollution is no longer just an issue of local toxicity.

Contribution of population increase to environmental change

The World Wildlife Fund for Nature has analyzed trends over the past three decades in the vitality and function of major categories of ecological systems, including freshwater ecosystems, marine ecosystems and forest ecosystems. Overall, the "Living Planet Index" has declined by 30 percent since 1970. Assessments by other researchers and international agencies approximately concur [7].

The three main determinants of human disruption of the environment are population size, the level of material wealth and consumption, and technology. The ongoing climate change debate illustrates well the relativities between the environmental effects of increases in population and consumption. Historically, during the twentieth Century, as population increased by just under fourfold the annual fossil fuel emissions of CO_2 increased twelvefold (Fig. 1.1). In 1995, the 20 percent of world population living in high-emission countries accounted for 63 percent of CO_2 emissions, while the lowest-emitting 20 percent of population contributed just 2 percent. Over the coming century the projected world population growth will contribute an estimated 35 percent of growth in CO_2 emissions, whereas economic growth would account for the remaining 65 percent.

If the world were to limit CO_2 buildup to a doubling of its pre-industrial concentration (i.e., from 275 to 550 ppm)—a level which climatologists think would be tolerable to most ecosystems—then the UN medium

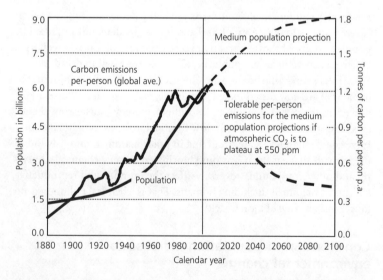

Fig. 1.1 Observed and projected time-trends in world population and globally averaged per-person carbon emissions (based on Ref. [22] with permission)

population projection of around ten billion by 2100 would allow per-person CO_2 emissions similar to those of the 1920–1930s. That is approximately two-thirds less than today's level of emissions. While this is a demanding task, much of the necessary technology exists to greatly reduce emissions without forfeiture of material standards of living. The real challenge is political—to transform current technologies and economic practice.

Overall, the larger potential threat is not from the increase in human numbers *per se* but from mildly environmentally disruptive humans becoming highly disruptive humans—in other words, from a "development" process that would generalise the patterns of production and consumption typical of today's rich countries. Current practices in rich countries are clearly *not* generalizable to a human population that is likely to reach 9–10 billion before 2100 and demand a higher average standard of living. The Netherlands now requires an estimated area fifteen times greater than its national size to support its population's way of life. It has been estimated that citizens of high-income countries today each require approximately 4–9 hectares of Earth's surface to provide the materials for their lifestyle and to absorb their wastes—while India's population gets by on one hectare per person. There will not be enough Earth to allow more than one hectare of "ecological footprint" per average-person when the world population reaches 9–10 billion [7].

Serious investment in the development and deployment of less environmentally disruptive technologies, and a much greater commitment to international equity, will be required if a smooth and timely transition to an ecologically sustainable world is to be achieved. Because rich countries remain the main source of new knowledge and new technologies, responsibility for finding paths to sustainability rests mainly with them. Minimizing the probabilities of long-term harm to health will be a major consideration and this issue is becoming the most important health-related aspect of the "population debate".

Global environmental changes and health: challenges for scientists

These historically unprecedented global environmental changes, pose a range of hazards to human health. Epidemiologists face some particular difficulties in assessing these environmentally induced risks. First, most incipient environmental changes have not yet exerted detectable impacts on human health; such impacts are likely to emerge over several decades [65]. Second, many of the causal pathways are of a complex and indirect kind—such as those likely to affect the transmission of vector-borne malaria and dengue fever, or the environmental impairment of agricultural yields and, hence, regional food insecurity. Third, as usual, the causality of disease in human populations is multivariate and this difficulty is further amplified by there being coexistent impacts of various environmental changes.

Detecting the early health impacts of global environmental changes will be difficult. Some clues, however, have begun to emerge—as with the northerly spread of tick-borne encephalitis in Sweden in association with winter warming over the past two decades [66]. Some of the recent spread of malaria and dengue fever may have been due to the climate change that has occurred over the past quarter-century, although there are other competing explanations. The persistence of approximately 800 million persons suffering from malnutrition may partly reflect the erosion of agroecosystem resources along with the adverse impacts of various large-scale environmental changes on photosynthesis, plant physiology and the occurrence of crop pests and diseases. Other evidence indicates that the tempo of extreme weather events and adverse human impacts has increased during the past decade. This probably reflects the climatic instability that characterizes global climate change [67].

Conclusion

The combination of rapid socioeconomic change, demographic change, and global environmental change, and their potential health impacts, requires a broad conception of the determinants of population health. A deficiency of social capital (social networks and civic institutions) adversely affects the prospects for health by predisposing to widened rich-poor gaps, and weakened public health systems. The large-scale loss of natural environmental capital—manifested as climate change, stratospheric ozone depletion, degradation of food-producing systems, depleted freshwater supplies, biodiversity loss, and spread of invasive species—is beginning to impair the biosphere's long-term capacity to sustain healthy human life.

Public health scientists and policy makers face unfamiliar challenges in addressing these broader dimensions of population health—while at the same time continuing to identify, quantify, and reduce the risks to health that result from specific, often local, social, behavioral, and environmental factors. This human-ecology perspective will broaden the theory and practice of public health, and will help integrate the consideration of health outcomes into decision-making in all policy sectors. The sustained good health of populations requires enlightened management of our social resources, economic relations, and of the natural world. There are win-win opportunities in this situation: many of today's public health issues have their roots in the same socioeconomic inequalities and imprudent consumption patterns that jeopardise the future sustainability of health.

A major contemporary challenge for public health and public policy at large, is to provide a satisfactory, healthy and equitable standard of living for current and future generations. This must include adequate food yields, clean water and energy, safe shelter, and functional ecosystems. Human-induced global environmental changes jeopardise our ability to meet this challenge. Human population health should be a key criterion of "sustainable development". Population health, in the medium- to longer-term is an indicator of how well we are managing our natural and social environments. History has shown that changes in human ecology and, in humankind's relationship to the natural environment shape the patterns of population health and survival. Application of this ecological perspective will be critical if a sustainable future is to be achieved [68,69]. These are great challenges for public health practitioners and researchers, challenges which most training programmes are not adequately addressing.

References

[1] Feachem RGA. Globalisation is good for your health, mostly. *BMJ* 2001; **323**: 504–6.

[2] Cornia GA. Globalisation and health: results and options. *Bull WHO* 2001; **79**: 834–41.

[3] McMichael AJ. Population, environment, disease, and survival: past patterns, uncertain futures. *Lancet* 2002; **359**: 1145–8.

[4] Beaglehole R, Bonita R. *Public Health at the Crossroads: Achievements and Prospects.* Cambridge: Cambridge University Press, 1997.

[5] Szreter S. The importance of social interventions in Britain's mortality decline c.1850–1914: a re-interpretaion of the role of public health. *Soc Hist Med* 1988; **1**: 1–37.

[6] Powles JW. Changes in disease patterns and related social trends. *Soc Sci Med* 1992; **35**: 377–87.

[7] McMichael AJ. *Human Frontiers, Environments and Disease: Past Patterns, Future Uncertainties.* Cambridge: Cambridge University Press, 2001.

[8] Acheson D. *Independent Inquiry into Inequalities in Health.* London: HM Stationery Office, 1998.

[9] Leon DA, Walt G (eds.). *Poverty, Inequality and Health*. Oxford: Oxford University Press, 2001.

[10] Legge D. Challenges of globalisation deserve better than simplistic polemics. *BMJ* 2002; **324**: 44.

[11] Butler CD. Inequality, global change and the sustainability of civilisation. *Glob Chge Humn Hlth* 2001; **1**: 156–72.

[12] Loomis D, Wing S. Is molecular epidemiology a germ theory for the end of the twentieth century? *Int J Epidemiol* 1990; **19**: 1–3.

[13] Pearce N. Traditional epidemiology, modern epidemiology, and public health. *Am J Public Health* 1996; **86**: 678–83.

[14] McMichael AJ. Prisoners of the proximate: epidemiology in an age of change. *Am J Epidemiol* 1999; **149**: 887–97.

[15] Eurowinter Group. Cold exposure and winter mortality from ischaemic heart disease, cerebrovascular disease, respiratory disease, and all causes in warm and cold regions of Europe. *Lancet* 1997; **349**: 1341–6.

[16] Wilkinson R. *Unhealthy Societies: The Afflictions of Inequality*. London: Routledge, 1996.

[17] Leon DA, Chenet L, Shkolnikov VM et al. Huge variation in Russian mortality rates 1984–94: artefact, alcohol, or what? *Lancet* 1997; **350**: 383–8.

[18] WHO. The World Health Report 1999: Making a difference. Geneva: WHO, 1999.

[19] Rees W. In: Crabbé P, Westra L, Holland A (eds.). *Implementing Ecological Integrity: Restoring Regional and Global Environmental and Human Health*. Dordrecht: Kluwer Academic Publishers, 2000.

[20] World Commission on Environment and Development. *Our Common Future*. Oxford: Oxford University Press, 1987.

[21] Report of the Commission on Macroeconomics and Health. *Macroeconomics and Health: Investing in Health for Economic Development*. Geneva: WHO, 2001.

[22] McMichael AJ, Powles JW. *Human population size, environment and health*. In: R Detels et al. (eds.). *Oxford Textbook of Public Health*, 4th edn. Oxford: Oxford University Press, 2002.

[23] Rotberg RI, Rabb TK. *Hunger and History*. Cambridge: Cambridge University Press, 1985.

[24] Hetzel BS. *The Story of Iodine Deficiency. An International Challenge in Nutrition*. Oxford: Oxford University Press, 1989.

[25] Trowell H, Burkitt D. *Western Disease: Their Emergence and Prevention*. London: Edward Arnold, 1981.

[26] Boyden S. *Western Civilization in Biological Perspective. Patterns in Biohistory*. Oxford: Oxford University Press, 1987.

[27] WHO. Diet, Nutrition and the Prevention of Chronic Diseases. *WHO, Technical Report Series 797*. Geneva: WHO, 1990.

[28] McMichael AJ, Beaglehole R. The changing global context of public health. *Lancet* 2000; **356**: 495–9.

[29] McMichael AJ. Human culture, ecological change and infectious disease: Are we experiencing history's Fourth Great Transition? *Ecosystem Health* 2001; 7: 107–15.

[30] McKeown T. *The Modern Rise of Population*. London: Arnold, 1976.

[31] Powles JW, Cumio F. Public health infrastructures and asociated knowledge as global public goods. In: R Beaglehole, R Smith, N Drager (eds.). *Global Public Goods for Health*. Oxford: Oxford University Press (in press).

[32] Powles JW, McMichael AJ. Human disease: Effects of economic development. In: *Encylopaedia of Life Sciences*. London: Macmillan, http://www.els.net, London: Nature Publishing Group, 2001.

[33] Caldwell JC. Routes to low mortality in poor countries. *Pop Dev Review* 1986; **12**: 171–220.

[34] Lee K. *Globalisation and Health: An introduction*. London: Palgrave, 2002.

[35] Yach D, Bettcher D. The globalization of public health, I: threats and opportunities. *Am J Public Health* 1998; **88**: 735–8.

[36] Yach D, Bettcher D. The globalization of public health, II: the convergence of self-interest and altruism. *Am J Public Health* 1998; **88**: 738–41.

[37] Gray J. *False Dawn: the Delusions of Global Capitalism*. London: Granta, 1998.

[38] Navarro V. Comment: whose globalization? *Am J Public Health* 1998; **88**: 742–3.

[39] Bassett M. Paper presented to *Ecological Society of South Africa*, annual scientific conference, East London, 23–25 February, 2000.

[40] World Bank. *The State in a Changing World: World Development Report 1997*. Oxford: Oxford University Press, 1997.

[41] Dollar D. Is globalisation good for your health? *Bull WHO* 2001; **79**: 827–33.

[42] Rodriguez F, Rodrik D. *Trade Policy and Economic Growth: a Skeptic's Guide to the Cross-National Evidence*. Mimeo, Harvard University, 1999.

[43] Milanovic B. True world income distribution, 1998 and 1993: First calculation based on household surveys alone. *Economic J* 2002; **112**: 51–92.

[44] Yach D, Bettcher D. Globalisation of tobacco industry influence and new global responses. *Tob Control* 2000; **9**: 206–16.

[45] Red Cross. *World Disasters Report*, 1998. New York: Oxford University Press, 1999.

[46] Levy BS, Sidel VW (eds.). *War and Public Health*. New York: Oxford University Press, 1997.

[47] McMichael AJ, Powles JW. Human numbers, environment, sustainability and health. *BMJ* 1999; **319**: 977–80.

[48] Daily G (ed.). *Nature's Services: Societal Dependence on Natural Ecosystems*. Washington, DC: Island Press, 1997.

[49] Loh J, Randers J, MacGillivray A, Kapos V, Jenkins M, Groombridge B, Cox
N. Living Planet Report, 1998. Gland, Switzerland: WWF International,
Switzerland; New Economics Foundation, London; World Conservation
Monitoring Centre, Cambridge; 1998.

[50] Last JM. Global environment, health and health services. In: JM Last,
RB Wallace (eds.) *Maxcy, Rosenau, Last. Public Health and Preventive
Medicine.* Norwalk, Connecticut: Appleton Lange, 1992, pp. 677–86.

[51] Intergovernmental Panel on Climate Change. Climate Change, 1995—The
Science of Climate Change: Contribution of Working Group I to the Second
Assessment Report of the Intergovernmental Panel on Climate Change. In:
JT Houghton, LG Meira Filho, BA Callander *et al.* (eds). Cambridge:
Cambridge University Press, UK, 1996.

[52] Climate Change Impacts Review Group (UK). The Potential Effects of
Climate Change in the United Kingdom. London: DETR, 1996.

[53] McMichael AJ, Haines A, Slooff R, Kovats RS (eds.). *Climate Change and
Human Health.* Geneva: WHO, 1996.

[54] McMichael AJ, Haines A. Global climate change: the potential effects on
health. *BMJ* 1997; **315**: 805–9.

[55] Martens WJM, Kovats RS, Nijhof S, de Vries P, Livermore MTJ,
Bradley D, Cox J, McMichael AJ. Climate change and future populations
at risk of malaria. *Global Environmental Change* 1999; **9** (Suppl):
S89–S107.

[56] UN Environment Programme. *Environmental Effects of Ozone Depletion.
1998 Assessment.* Lausanne: Elsevier, 1998.

[57] Slaper H., Velders GJM, Daniel JS, de Gruijl FR, van der Leun, JC. Estimates
of ozone depletion and skin cancer incidence to examine the Vienna
Convention achievements. *Nature* 1996, **384**: 256–8.

[58] Myers N. Biodiversity's genetic library. In: GC Daily (ed.). Nature's Services:
Societal Dependence on Natural Ecosystems. Washington DC: Island Press,
1997.

[59] Epstein PR. Weeds bring disease to the east African waterways. *Lancet* 1998;
351: 577.

[60] Pimentel D, Harvey C, Resosudarmo P et al. Environmental and
economic costs of soil erosion and conservation benefits. *Science* 1995; **267**:
1117–22.

[61] World Resources Institute. World Resources 1998–1999. *Environment and
Health.* Oxford: Oxford University Press, 1998.

[62] Food and Agricultural Organization. State of the World's Fisheries, 1995.
Rome, Italy: FAO, 1995.

[63] Parry M, C. Rosenzweig, A. Iglesias, G. Fischer, M.T.J. Livermore. Climate
change and global food security: a new assessment. *Global Environmental
Change* 1999; **9** (Suppl): S51–S67.

[64] UK Meteorology Office, UK Department of Environment, Transport and Regions. Climate Change and Its Impacts. ISBN 0 86180 346 9. London: Met Office Communications, 1998.

[65] Kovats RS, Campbell-Lendrum, McMichael AJ, Woodward A, Cox J StH. Early effects of climate change: do they include changes in vector-borne disease? *Phil Trans Roy Soc Lond B*, 2001; 356: 1–12.

[66] Lindgren E, Gustafson R. Tick-borne encephalitis in Sweden and climate change. *Lancet* 2001; **358**: 16–18.

[67] Intergovernmental Panel on Climate Change, Climate Change 2000, Report of WGII. Cambridge: Cambridge University Press, 2001.

[68] McMichael AJ, Smith KR, Corvalan C. The Sustainability Transition: A new challenge. *Bull WHO* 2000; **78**: 1067.

[69] Kates RW, Clark WC, Corell R et al. Environment and development. Sustainability Science. *Science* 2001; **292**: 641–2.

Chapter 2

Global health status at the beginning of the twenty-first century

Ruth Bonita and Colin D Mathers

Introduction

The impressive improvements in health status worldwide over the last century are a cause for celebration. Public health professionals can feel proud of their contribution to these achievements even as they appreciate the complexity of the underlying driving forces, many of which lie outside traditional public health work. However, satisfaction must be tempered by several concerns. Firstly, the health improvements have not been shared equally and health inequalities among and within countries remain entrenched. Secondly, the fragility of health gains has repeatedly been demonstrated in response, for example, to economic and social changes and civil disruption. Thirdly, and as we have seen in Chapter 1, the global health situation is a complex and a challenging mixture of old and new health problems.

These factors suggest that from a global perspective, sustainable and equitable health advancement is not yet secure especially as the economic disparities between countries continue to grow. This chapter provides an overview of global health status and highlights the importance of capturing, with a range of new measures, the health transformations that are taking place in the context of continuing global change.

Measures of health status

Mortality, risk of death and life expectancy

The best known health status measure continues to be cause of death based on the death certificate. The system of classifying causes of death developed by William Farr 150 years ago still forms the basis of the International Classification of Diseases, now in its tenth version. This provides an invaluable source of information on patterns of death and trends over time. Unfortunately, complete cause specific death registration data are routinely available for only a minority of the world's countries. Less than one third of the world's population is adequately covered by national vital registration systems and there is a wide regional variation ranging from 80 percent population coverage in the European region to less than 5 percent population coverage in the Eastern Mediterranean and African regions of the World Health Organization (WHO). However, complete or incomplete vital registration data together with sample registration systems now cover 74 percent of global mortality. Survey data and indirect demographic techniques provide information on levels of child and adult mortality for the remaining 26 percent of estimated global mortality. Data sources and methods are described in more detail elsewhere; these data are of variable quality and there are still a few countries for which no recent data on levels of adult or child mortality are available [1].

While much attention has been directed at obtaining data on children under five and maternal mortality (for example from extensive child mortality surveys such as the Demographic Health Surveys (DHS) or the Multiple Indicator Cluster Survey (MICS) programme of UNICEF), the most serious information gap now is for adult mortality. Fortunately, considerable effort has gone into developing alternatives to national routine death certification. For example, in China, provincial authorities have provided death data on a routine basis for the past decade from a nationally representative system of 145 disease surveillance points (DSP) covering 1 percent of the total Chinese population [2]. At each surveillance point, a team that includes a physician, investigates each death using medical records and interviews with family members to assign a cause of death. Data on the age, sex and cause of 50,000–60,000 deaths are recorded each year. Periodic evaluations of the DSP data by re-surveying households at random suggest a level of underreporting of deaths of about 15 percent [2]. In addition, there has been substantial improvement in recent years in the Vital Registration System of the Ministry of Health in China, and this now provides additional useful information for China. Data on the age, sex and cause of 725,000 deaths are collected annually from the vital registration system operated by the Ministry of Health, covering a population of 121 million (sixty-six million in urban areas, fifty-five million in rural areas). While the data are not representative of mortality conditions throughout China, they are useful for suggesting trends in mortality, given the number of deaths covered, and also provide valuable information on cause of death patterns. A third source of data on mortality in China is an annual one per 1000 household survey which asks about deaths in the past 12 months [2]. From these three low-cost information sources, it has been possible to extrapolate to the national level and contribute to estimates of global patterns and causes of death.

Similar attempts have been made in India where, to compensate for a poor civil registration system, the Sample Registration System has successfully collected data on rural mortality and fertility since 1964–65 through continuous recording by resident enumerators as well as retrospective half-yearly population surveys. Data are collected on vital events in 4,436 rural and 2,235 urban sampling units with a population of about six million people covering almost all States and Territories. Comparison of these data with other survey and demographic estimates suggest that underreporting of child deaths is minimal and of adult deaths is around 15 percent. The Medical Certificate of Cause of Death (MCCD) provides information for deaths in urban India. A high coverage of all deaths (estimated at 95 percent) has been achieved using these multiple approaches [3].

An alternative to the medically certified death certificate, the verbal autopsy, has also been shown to be economical and useful in improving the quality of cause of death information where health workers have minimal training [4–6]. Verbal autopsy information is, however, still far from ideal, and of relatively limited use for certain groups of causes of death with similar symptom patterns. WHO is exploring the use of verbal autopsy in population surveys to identify injury deaths, particularly deaths related to war and civil conflict [7].

These multiple sources have been used by WHO, together with information derived from specific epidemiological studies, to estimate life tables and cause of death patterns for all regions of the world [8,9]. In countries with a substantial HIV epidemic, separate estimates were made of the numbers and distributions of deaths due to HIV/AIDS and these deaths incorporated into the life table estimates [10].

Disability and health status measures

While risk of death is the simplest comparable measure of health status for populations, there has been increasing interest in describing, measuring and comparing health states of populations. These have been conceptualized in two main ways: in terms of disability and handicap, and in terms of multidimensional health profiles [11]. In the latter approach, a health state is a multi-dimensional attribute of an individual that reflects his or her level in the various domains of health. Thus, a health state differs from pathology, risk factors or etiology, and from health service encounters or interventions. Describing health states within and between populations is a central challenge in undertaking the measurement of health.

The WHO International Classification of Impairments, Disabilities, and Handicaps (ICIDH) defined *disability* as any restriction or lack of ability (resulting from an impairment) to perform an activity in the manner or within the range considered normal for a human being; and *handicap* as the social disadvantage resulting from an impairment or a disability that limits or prevents the fulfillment of a normal role [12]. The second revision of the ICIDH, now called the International Classification of Functioning, Disability and Health (or ICF) replaces the ICIDH concepts of disability and handicap by the concepts of *capacity* and *performance* and applies these constructs to a single list of tasks and activities [13]. The term *disability* is now used broadly to refer to departures from good or ideal health in any of the important domains of health.

Existing disability and health state measurement instruments have differed considerably in their content in an attempt to arrive at a set of domains that covers the universe of disability or health adequately. However, problems with comparability of self-report health and disability data relate not only to differences in survey questions and methods, but more fundamentally to unmeasured differences in expectations and norms for health [14,15]. For example, the level of mobility described as "moderate limitations" may differ across different cultures, across socioeconomic groups within a society, across age groups or between men and women.

Comparability is fundamental to the use of survey results for measuring population health but has been under-emphasized in instrument development. In 2000–2001, WHO carried out a Multi-Country Survey Study in over sixty countries and developed a health module based on selected domains of the ICF and used a set of six core domains for measuring health states: pain, affect, cognition, mobility, self-care and usual activities (including household and work related activities) [16]. The WHO survey program has at its first objective the assessment of health in different domains for nationally representative adult population samples in a way that is comparable across populations. To do this, the survey includes case vignettes and some measured tests on selected domains that are intended to calibrate the description that respondents provide of their own health. WHO has developed statistical methods for correcting biases in self-reported health using these data [17].

Responses for sixty-three surveys in fifty-five countries from the WHO Multi-Country Survey study were used to estimate the true prevalence of different states of health by age and sex. The sampled populations were adults aged eighteen years and over. Just over one-half (thirty-four) of the surveys were household interview surveys, two were telephone surveys, and the remainder postal surveys. Thirty-five of the surveys were carried out in thirty-one European countries, twenty-two surveys in nineteen developing countries, and the remaining six in Canada, United States, Australia and New Zealand.

Summary measures combining mortality and morbidity

The epidemiological transition, characterized by a progressive rise in the average age of death in virtually all populations across the globe, has necessitated a serious reconsideration of how the health of populations is measured. Average life expectancy at birth is becoming increasingly uninformative in many populations where, because of the nonlinear relationship between age-specific mortality and the life expectancy index, significant declines in death rates at older ages have produced only relatively modest increases in life expectancy at birth. Such considerations are critical for the planning and provision of health and social services, as resources are now devoted to reducing the incidence of conditions that cause ill health but not death.

Separate measures of survival and of health status among survivors, while useful inputs into the health policy debate, need to be combined in some fashion if the goal is to provide a single, holistic measure of overall population health. Two classes of health status measures have been developed that combine mortality and morbidity into a single index: health gaps and health expectancies [18]. Both these types of summary measure use time as a common currency for years of life lived in various states of health and for time lost due to premature mortality.

Burden of disease and health gap measures

The Global Burden of Disease (GBD) project developed a new summary measure that combines the impact of premature mortality with that of disability and captures the impact on populations of important nonfatal disabling conditions [19]. Disability adjusted life years (DALYs) combine time lost through premature death and time lived with disability. One DALY can be thought of as one lost year of "healthy" life and the measured disease burden is the gap between a population's health status and that of a normative reference population (with life expectancy at birth of 82.5 years for females and 80.0 years for males). The DALY is a generalization of the well known mortality gap measure Years of Potential Life Lost (YPLL) to include lost good health. It also provides a way to link information at the population level on disease causes and occurrence to information on both short-term and long-term health outcomes, including impairments, disability and death. In this measure, as in YPLL, causes of death that occur early in life are weighted more heavily than those that occur later in life and do not take into account competing risks [20] but rather measure years lost against a normative standard.

WHO is now undertaking a new assessment of the Global Burden of Disease (GBD) for the year 2000 based on an extensive analysis of mortality data for all regions of the world together with systematic reviews of epidemiological studies and population health surveys. These revisions draw on a wide range of data sources, and various methods have been developed to reconcile often fragmented and partial estimates of epidemiological parameters that are available from different studies [21].

The GBD project in general, and the DALY measure in particular, have stimulated considerable debate, in part due to the limitations of the basic data, the extrapolations from these data to entire regions, the assumptions that are needed for these estimates, and indeed the justification for the project [22–24]. The greatest degree of uncertainty relates to the sub-Saharan estimates because of the scarcity of epidemiological data [25]. The GBD projects have as one of their major objectives an assessment of all causes of disease and injury burden. Otherwise, limitations in the evidence base for certain causes or regions translate to "no burden" rather than the best achievable uncertain estimates of burden and health decision makers would be presented with a misleading picture. Where the evidence is uncertain, incomplete or even nonexistent, the GBD 2000 attempts us to make the best possible inferences based on the knowledge base that is available, and to assess the uncertainty in the resulting estimates. This has generated controversy among epidemiologists who are more used to reporting only assessments with narrow uncertainty intervals primarily based on sampling error.

The social values and disability weights incorporated into the DALY have also attracted criticism. Some critics have argued against the use of age weights that give lower value to years of life lived in early childhood and older ages [26,27] and some recent national burden of disease studies have used time discounting but not age weights [28]. However, the most persistent criticisms have been that burden of disease analysis may result in incorrect policy decisions, for example, that the end result could be to penalise the poor and elderly people by according priority to young and middle ages [29] or to fuel competition for resources between advocates for communicable disease and noncommunicable disease prevention strategies when many of the global forces underlying these disease categories are similar [30,31].

These criticisms stem from a concern that priorities for health action might be set solely on the basis of the magnitude of burden of disease. However, the different diseases, injuries and risk factors contributing to loss of health are important factors as, are cost-effectiveness of interventions and other information relating to equity and social values in informing health policy in relation to the potentials for improvement of population health [24].

Health expectancy measures

Another form of summary measure of population health, the health expectancy, has been used since the 1970s to report on average levels of population health. Disability-free life expectancy (DFLE) was calculated and reported for many countries in the 1980s and 1990s [32,33]. Unfortunately, DFLE estimates based on self-reported health status information are not comparable across countries due to differences in survey instruments and cultural differences in reporting of health [34].

In its World Health Report 2000, WHO for the first time reported on the average levels of population health for its 191 member countries using disability-adjusted life expectancy (DALE) which measures the equivalent number of years of life expected to be lived in full health [9,35]. Updated estimates of healthy life expectancy for the year 2000 were published in the World Health Report 2001 using improved methods and incorporating cross-population comparable survey data from sixty-three surveys in fifty-five countries [9]. To better reflect the inclusion of all states of health in the calculation of healthy life expectancy, the name of the indicator used to measure healthy life expectancy was changed from DALE to healthy life expectancy (HALE).

Some commentators have argued that the data demands and complexity of the calculations make healthy life expectancy an impractical measure for use as a summary measure of population health [36]. Although the concept of healthy life expectancy is relatively simple to understand, health encompasses multiple domains and mortality risks, and with the additional requirement to ensure comparability of estimates across countries, any acceptable methods used to compute healthy life expectancy will inevitably be complex.

An overview of global health status

Mortality patterns

WHO estimates that almost fifty-six million people died in 2000, 10.9 million (or nearly 20 percent) of whom were children less than five years of age [9].

Of these child deaths, 99.3 percent occurred in developing countries. Almost 70 percent of deaths in developed countries occur beyond age seventy, compared with about 30 percent in developing countries. A key point is the comparatively high numbers of deaths in developing countries at young adult ages (15–59 years). Just over 30 percent of all deaths in developing countries occur at these ages, compared with 15 percent in richer regions. This vast premature adult mortality in developing countries is of major public health concern.

The variations across regions of the world in the probability of premature death, for example, between birth and five years and between age fifteen and sixty years, give one indication of the potential for health improvement. The twentyfold variation in infant mortality between different regions of the world is largely due to communicable diseases, malnutrition and poverty (Fig. 2.1). In contrast, the probability of death in adults aged between fifteen years and sixty years is due mostly to noncommunicable diseases and injury, except in India and sub-Saharan Africa.

The probability of premature death varies widely between regions. For example, for men in eastern European countries (FSE), the proportion is similar to that of men in developing regions of Asia and the Middle East

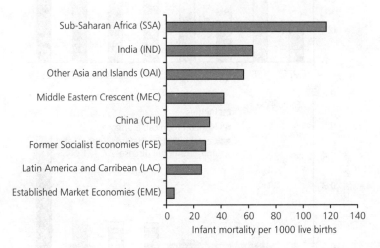

Fig. 2.1 Global variation in infant mortality rates, 2000

Note: Regional groupings are those used in the Global Burden of Disease Study [19]. EME includes Western Europe, North America, Japan, Australia and New Zealand, FSE includes the former socialist countries of Eastern Europe and Central Asia, OAI includes Asian and Pacific countries apart from India, China, Japan, Australia and New Zealand. MEC includes Middle Eastern countries and North African countries

(Fig. 2.2). Men in these regions are three times more likely to die prematurely than men in western industrialized populations represented in the graph by established market economies (EME). The variation in proportion of women dying prematurely in these regions is much less dramatic, except for the differences between EME and SSA.

Developing countries themselves are a very heterogeneous group in terms of mortality. A contrast between China (with more than one-sixth of the world's population) and Africa (with one-tenth of global population) illustrates the extreme diversity in health conditions among developing regions. Less than 10 percent of deaths in China occur below age five compared with

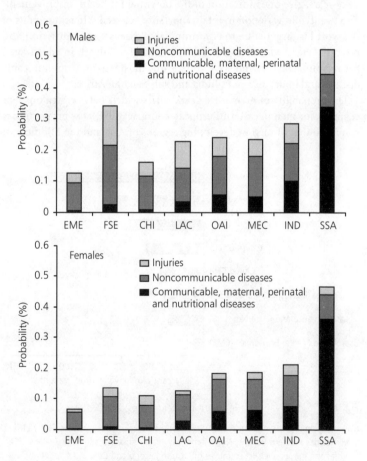

Fig. 2.2 Probability of death between ages fifteen and sixty years, by sex and region, 2000 (refer to Fig. 2.1 for explanation of regions)

40 percent in Africa. Conversely, 45 percent of deaths in China occur beyond age seventy, whereas only 10 percent in Africa do.

Of the fifty-six million deaths in 2000, 32.8 million or 59 percent were due to noncommunicable diseases, which killed twice as many people as communicable, maternal, perinatal, and nutritional causes combined (17.8 million, or 31 percent of all causes). Injuries killed a further 5.1 million people in 2000, almost one in ten of the world's total deaths. The relative importance of these causes varies markedly across regions. Thus in Africa, only about one in five deaths are due to noncommunicable diseases, compared with more than four out of five in industrialized countries. Two-thirds of deaths in Latin America and close to three-quarters in the developing regions of the Asia and the Western Pacific are due to noncommunicable disease reflecting the relatively advanced stage of the epidemiological transition achieved in these populations.

Life expectancy

Life expectancy at birth ranges from 81.4 years for women in the established market economies of Western Europe, North American, Japan, Australia and New Zealand down to 48.1 years for men in sub-Saharan Africa (Fig. 2.3). This is a 1.7-fold difference in total life expectancy across major regions of the globe. Overall, for the entire population of the world, average life expectancy at birth in 2000 was 65.5 years, an increase of six years over the last two decades. As shown in Fig.2.3, life expectancy increased during the 1990s for most regions of the world, with the notable exception of Africa and the former Soviet countries of Eastern Europe. In the latter case, male and female life expectancies at birth declined by 3.2 years and 2.7 years, respectively, over the 10-year period between 1990 and 2000.

The top ten disease and injury causes of death in the year 2000 for developed countries and developing countries are shown in Table 2.1. In developed countries, ischaemic heart disease and cerebrovascular disease (stroke) are together responsible for 36 percent of mortality, and death rates are higher for men than women. This proportion has decreased slightly from 38 percent in 1990. The increase in cardiovascular mortality in Eastern European countries has been offset by continuing declines in many other developed countries. Lung cancer is the third leading cause of death, again with a nearly 3-fold male excess. Another largely tobacco-related cause, chronic obstructive lung disease, is the fifth leading cause of death, accounting for 3 percent of deaths in developed countries. Suicide accounts for nearly 2 percent of deaths in developed countries, a proportion that has remained unchanged since 1990. Road traffic

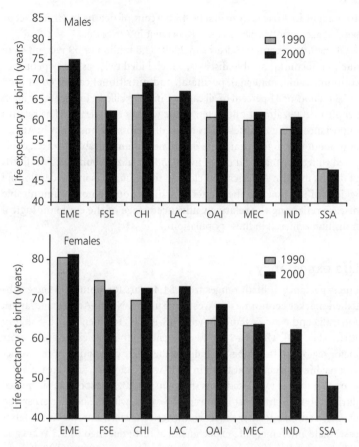

Fig. 2.3 Gains in life expectancy at birth from 1990 to 2000, by sex and region (refer to Fig. 2.1 for explanation of regions)

accidents are no longer in the top ten causes of mortality, as there has been a decline in death rates due to road traffic accidents of nearly 30 percent since 1990.

The leading causes of mortality are very different in developing countries (Table 2.1). While the two leading causes of death in 2000 are ischaemic heart disease and cerebrovascular disease, six of the top ten causes of death in developing countries are infectious and perinatal causes. Acute lower respiratory infectious (primarily pneumonia) are the second leading cause of death (60 percent of these among children aged under five). HIV/AIDS is the fourth leading cause of death for developing

Table 2.1 Ten leading causes of death, developed and developing countries[1], 2000

	Percent of total deaths	Male to female ratio
Developed countries		
1 Ischaemic heart disease	22.6	1.0
2 Cerebrovascular disease	13.7	0.6
3 Trachea, bronchus, lung cancers	4.5	2.7
4 Lower respiratory infections	3.7	0.9
5 Chronic obstructive pulmonary disease	3.1	1.5
6 Colon and rectum cancers	2.6	1.0
7 Stomach cancer	1.9	1.5
8 Self-inflicted injuries	1.9	3.6
9 Diabetes mellitus	1.7	0.7
10 Breast cancer	1.6	1.9
Developing countries		
1 Ischaemic heart disease	9.1	1.2
2 Cerebrovascular disease	8.0	1.2
3 Lower respiratory infections	7.7	1.0
4 HIV/AIDS	6.9	1.0
5 Perinatal conditions	5.6	1.1
6 Chronic obstructive pulmonary disease	5.0	1.1
7 Diarrhoeal diseases	4.9	1.2
8 Tuberculosis	3.7	1.6
9 Malaria	2.6	0.9
10 Road traffic accidents	2.5	2.8

[1] Developed countries include Established Market Economies (EME) & Former Socialist Economies (FSE).

countries in 2000, accounting for 2.9 million deaths. More than 80 percent of these deaths occurred in Africa, making HIV the leading cause of death in this region, claiming almost one in four deaths. Chronic obstructive lung disease kills more people (1.5 million) in the Western Pacific Region (primarily China) than anywhere else in the world, with 60 percent of global mortality from the disease occurring there.

Other leading causes of death in developing countries include two major causes of childhood mortality, perinatal conditions and diarrhoeal diseases, which claim 2.4 and 2.1 million lives each year, respectively, followed by TB (1.6 million), malaria and road traffic accidents. While death rates due to perinatal conditions have declined slightly compared with 1990, death rates due to diarrhoeal diseases have declined substantially, with an estimated 2.9 million deaths in 1990 [9].

There were an estimated 1.2 million lung cancer deaths in 2000, an increase of nearly 30 percent in the ten years from 1990. Of the 6.9 million cancer deaths estimated to have occurred in 2000, one in six (18 percent) were due to lung cancer alone and of these, three-quarters occurred among men. Stomach cancer, which until recently was the leading site of cancer mortality worldwide, has been declining in all parts of the world where trends can be reliably assessed and now causes 744,000 deaths each year, or about two-thirds as many as lung cancer. Liver cancer is the third leading site, with 626,000 deaths a year, more than half (56 percent) of which are estimated to occur in the Western Pacific Region.

On average, HIV/AIDS has reduced life expectancy for sub-Saharan Africans by six years in 2000. The largest impact has been in Zimbabwe, Botswana and Namibia, where male and female life expectancies would be around twenty years higher if there were no deaths due to HIV/AIDS.

Disability and health status

The recent results from the WHO Multi-Country Survey provide the only measures of disability and health status available which are comparable across countries [17,37]. Figure 2.4 summarizes the average severity-weighted prevalences by age and sex for surveys in the EME (twenty-eight surveys), FSE (eleven surveys) and developing countries (twenty-one surveys). Figure 2.4 shows arithmetic averages of age-specific prevalences for surveys, not population-weighted estimates for regions, and is intended only to illustrate the broad patterns of health status by age, sex, and region. The severity-weighted prevalence of health states less than full health increases with age as expected, and is higher for developing countries than the established market economies. What is surprising are the high prevalences for the former socialist economies of Eastern Europe, higher than prevalences for the developing regions. These high prevalences are influenced by high levels of anxiety and depression, even after adjustment

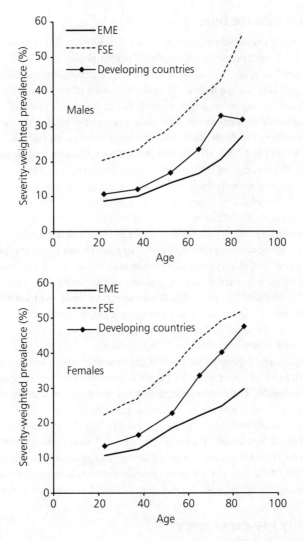

Fig. 2.4 Prevalence of health related status in developed (EME and FSE) and developing countries

for cross-population differences in the use of response categories in the WHO survey module using vignettes to define fixed levels of affect. Health status in women is generally somewhat worse than in men at most ages, except in Eastern Europe.

Global disease burden in 2000

The leading causes of DALYs worldwide for the year 2000 are shown in Table 2.2. Lower respiratory infections, perinatal conditions, HIV/AIDS and unipolar depressive disorders are the three leading causes of DALYs for males and females combined. The global burden of diarrhoeal diseases, conditions arising in the perinatal period, and congenital anomalies have all declined, from a combined total of 16.3 percent of total DALYs in 1990 to 12.6 percent in 2000. Reflecting the huge increase in HIV incidence between 1990 and 2000, HIV/AIDS has leapt from the 28th leading cause of DALYS (0.8 percent) in 1990 to third leading cause (6.1 percent) in 2000.

HIV/AIDS is actually the leading cause of the disease burden in women globally. The total DALYs are similar in magnitude for men and women, with the rankings reflecting a higher total burden for men from other causes. A more important sex difference is for depression, which is the fourth leading cause of disease burden in women but ranks seventh for men. Road traffic accidents are a leading cause of overall disease and injury burden in men (4.0 percent) but not in women (1.5 percent). Indeed, when DALYs rather than deaths are considered, the public health importance of injuries becomes more apparent. In parts of South Asia, Eastern Europe and the Western Pacific, 20 percent or more of the entire disease and injury burden is due to injuries alone.

Table 2.2 also highlights the marked contrast in epidemiological patterns between rich and poor regions of the world, even more so than comparisons based on deaths. Thus in the more developed countries, the share of disease burden due to communicable, maternal, perinatal and nutritional conditions is typically around 5 percent, compared with 70–75 percent in Africa (not shown). Specifically, the leading causes of disease burden in Africa in 2000 were HIV/AIDS (20.6 percent), malaria (10.1 percent) and acute lower respiratory infections (8.6 percent), compared with ischaemic heart disease, depression, alcohol dependence and stroke in the developed countries.

Healthy life expectancy

Overall, global healthy life expectancy (HALE) at birth for males and females combined has been estimated to be 56.0 years in 2000, 9.0 years lower than total life expectancy at birth of 65.0 years [38]. Global HALE at birth for females is just over two years greater than that for men (Table 2.3). In comparison, total life expectancy at birth for females is almost four years higher than that for males. Regional healthy life expectancies at birth in 2000 ranged from a low of thirty-nine years for African men and women to a high of almost seventy-two years for women in the low mortality countries

AN OVERVIEW OF GLOBAL HEALTH STATUS | 39

Table 2.2 Ten leading causes of DALYs globally and in developed and developing countries,[1] global estimates for 2000

All countries	Percent total DALYs	Developed countries[1]	Percent total DALYs	Developing countries	Percent total DALYs
1 Lower respiratory infections	6.4	1 Unipolar depressive disorders	8.8	1 Lower respiratory infections	6.8
2 Perinatal conditions	6.2	2 Ischaemic heart disease	6.7	2 Perinatal conditions	6.7
3 HIV/AIDS	6.1	3 Alcohol use disorders	5.4	3 HIV/AIDS	6.6
4 Unipolar depressive disorders	4.4	4 Cerebrovascular disease	4.9	4 Meningitis	4.6
5 Diarrhoeal diseases	4.2	5 Alzheimer and other dementias	4.3	5 Diarrhoeal diseases	4.6
6 Ischaemic heart disease	3.8	6 Road traffic accidents	3.1	6 Unipolar depressive disorders	4.0
7 Cerebrovascular disease	3.1	7 Lung cancer	3.0	7 Ischaemic heart disease	3.5
8 Road traffic accidents	2.8	8 Osteoarthritis	2.7	8 Malaria	3.0
9 Malaria	2.7	9 COPD[2]	2.5	9 Cerebrovascular disease	2.9
10 Tuberculosis	2.4	10 Hearing loss, adult onset	2.5	10 Road traffic accidents	2.8

[1] As published in the World Health Report 2001 [9]. Developed countries include Established Market Economies (EME) and Former Socialist Economies (FSE).
[2] Chronic Obstructive Pulmonary Disease.

Table 2.3 Life expectancy (LE), healthy life expectancy (HALE), and lost healthy years as percent of total LE (LHE percent), at birth and at age sixty, by sex and region, 2000

Region[1]	Females			Males			Female-male difference		
	HALE (years)	LE (years)	LHE percent (percent)	HALE (years)	LE (years)	LHE percent (percent)	HALE (years)	LE (years)	LHE percent (percent)
At birth									
EME	72.0	81.2	11.4	68.0	75.1	9.5	4.0	6.1	1.9
FSE	61.0	72.2	15.5	54.0	62.9	14.2	7.0	9.3	1.3
LAC	61.8	73.7	16.1	58.0	67.0	13.4	3.8	6.7	2.7
MEC	55.9	69.4	19.5	56.4	66.1	14.7	−0.6	3.3	4.8
IND	51.7	62.7	17.5	52.2	59.8	12.7	−0.5	2.9	4.8
CHI	63.3	73.0	13.2	60.9	68.9	11.6	2.4	4.1	1.6
OAI	57.5	67.6	15.0	56.2	63.9	12.2	1.3	3.6	2.8
SSA	38.9	48.8	20.3	39.5	47.0	15.9	−0.6	1.9	4.4
World	57.0	67.2	15.1	54.9	62.7	12.5	2.1	4.5	2.7

Region[1]	Females			Males			Female-male difference		
	HALE (years)	LE (years)	LHE percent (percent)	HALE (years)	LE (years)	LHE percent (percent)	HALE (years)	LE (years)	LHE percent (percent)
At age sixty									
EME	18.8	24.2	22.4	15.9	19.9	19.8	2.9	4.4	2.6
FSE	13.0	18.9	31.5	9.6	14.6	34.2	3.3	4.3	−2.7
LAC	14.1	20.8	32.2	12.3	17.5	29.9	1.8	3.3	2.2
MEC	10.3	18.0	42.4	10.4	16.1	35.5	0.0	1.9	6.9
IND	10.9	17.7	38.6	9.9	14.6	32.4	1.0	3.1	6.2
CHI	14.3	20.4	29.8	11.8	16.6	29.0	2.5	3.8	0.8
OAI	12.9	19.0	32.2	11.1	15.9	29.8	1.7	3.1	2.4
SSA	8.3	15.8	47.3	8.3	13.9	40.2	0.0	1.9	7.1
World	14.1	20.2	30.3	11.9	16.7	28.3	2.2	3.6	2.0

[1] Refer to Fig. 2.1 for definitions of regions.

of Western Europe, North America and the Western Pacific region. This is almost a 2-fold difference in healthy life expectancy between major regional populations of the world. The difference between HALE and total life expectancy is LHE (healthy life expectancy "lost" due to disability). The equivalent "lost" healthy years range from 20 percent (of total life expectancy at birth) in women in Africa to less than 10 percent in men in low mortality countries.

In countries with HALE at birth of forty-five years or lower, male and female HALE are almost the same (Table 2.3). These countries are almost entirely African countries, but include the Lao People's Republic, Haiti and Nepal. There are a number of countries with HALE around fifty years, where female HALE at birth is actually lower than male HALE. These countries are mostly in Africa and the Eastern Mediterranean region, but also include Afghanistan, Pakistan and Bangladesh. For other countries with HALE at birth of greater than fifty years, female HALE is generally higher than male HALE, though the gap is lower than for total life expectancy. Similar patterns are apparent for the male-female gap in healthy life expectancy at age sixty, although the male-female reversal in Eastern Mediterranean countries no longer occurs.

Regional healthy life expectancies at age sixty in 2000 ranged from a low of 8.3 years for men and women in Africa to a high of around nineteen years for women in low-mortality countries. The equivalent "lost" healthy years at age sixty are a higher percentage of remaining life expectancy, due to the higher prevalence of disability at older ages. These range from around 40 to 50 percent in sub-Saharan Africa to around 20 percent in developed countries (Table 2.3).

The female-male difference in healthy life expectancy is greatest for Eastern European countries, at 7.0 years. In Eastern European countries, healthy life expectancy is 60.6 years for women, five years below the European average, but just 50.3 years for men, 9.6 years below the European average. This is one of the widest sex gaps in the world and reflects the sharp increase in adult male mortality in the early 1990s. The most common explanation is the high incidence of male alcohol abuse, which led to high rates of accidents, violence and cardiovascular disease. From 1987 to 1994, the risk of premature death increased by 70 percent for Russian males [39,40]. Between 1994 and 1998, life expectancy improved for males, but has declined significantly again in the last three years. Similar rates exist for other countries of the former Soviet Union. This pattern is explored in greater detail in Chapter 5.

Figure 2.5 shows average healthy life expectancy at birth for 191 countries (with 95 percent uncertainty intervals), plotted against income per capita

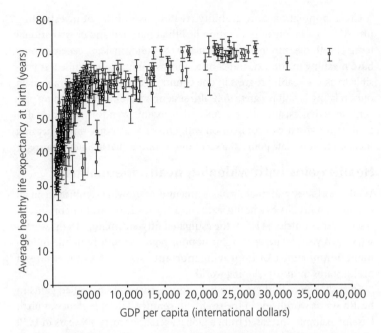

Fig. 2.5 Healthy life expectancy at birth versus Gross Domestic Product (GDP) per capita in international dollars (purchasing power parity conversion), 191 countries, 2000

(Gross Domestic Product measured in international dollars using purchasing power parity conversion rates) on a logarithmic scale. The error bars show estimated 95 percent uncertainty ranges for HALE at birth, reflecting uncertainty in life table parameters, health state prevalences and valuations. Country-specific estimates of male and female HALE and total life expectancy at birth and at age sixty, together with 95 percent uncertainty ranges, are published in the World Health Report 2001[9].

Discussion

Advances in measuring health states and disability

The new methods used in the WHO Multi-country Household Survey Study have increased the comparability of self-report data across countries and are a major step forward in the use of self-reported data on health. Building on this experience, WHO is developing improved health status measurement techniques for a World Health Survey to be carried out in 2002.

Cross-population comparability creates possibilities of investigating broad determinants of population health at national and cross-national level. Health measurements, particularly for policy makers, generally only have meaning in context, and context means comparison. While it is possible to assess health progress in one country using time-comparable data only, relating health progress to health system interventions, including prevention activities, and other social and economic trends is extremely difficult in the absence of comparison with other populations, simply because there is only one data point (the set of interventions that actually occurred).

Health gains with widening health inequalities

While morbidity and disability assessment is of growing significance in all countries, mortality as a health status measure is still of great importance in the poorer countries [41]. Of the estimated fifty-six million deaths worldwide each year, 80 percent occur in poor regions reinforcing the fundamental importance of improving mortality statistics as a measure of health status in the developing world.

Overall, however, there have been impressive and unrivalled gains in health status worldwide in the twentieth century. Life expectancy at birth has, for example, increased from a global average of forty-six years in 1950 to sixty-five years in 2000; even in the two decades since 1978, life expectancy has increased three years for men (reaching sixty-three years in 2000) and two years for women (reaching sixty-seven years in 2000). However, many populations in poor countries, and even a few in wealthy countries, still have life expectancies and disease profiles typical of European countries a century ago. Life expectancy at birth in the most developed countries at over eighty years is double that of the most disadvantaged countries. The relative disparity in years in life expectancy at birth among regions has hardly improved over the last half-century. In the twenty-year period from 1978, life expectancy at birth in high-income European countries increased by five years from seventy-three years. In the low and middle-income countries, life expectancy remained static at sixty-eight years. In almost all countries, women have longer life expectancy than men, with the notable exception of countries in the Eastern Mediterranean region and North Africa.

Life expectancies at birth, however, may disguise smaller differences in the duration of later life; for people in poor countries who survive to reach middle age, life expectancy begins to approach that of people in developed countries, but with the potential of earlier functional ageing among survivors. Regional life expectancy data also hide important and sobering national and within country differences and trends. For example, within the United States, the racial differences are large with Afro-American men having a life expectancy at birth up to twenty years lower than white men [42]. Within the Eastern Mediterranean region of the WHO, life expectancy at birth of women in Djibouti is twenty-eight years less than the life expectancy of women in Cyprus.

Another important feature of life expectancy patterns within countries is the powerful inverse association with social status. The health gains of the past decade have mainly benefited the better off [43,44]. While the best data are from the United Kingdom, the same pattern has been observed in all countries where suitable data are available, including the former socialist countries of Eastern Europe [45].

The extent of the global inequalities in health is illustrated by the large variations in child (under five years of age) mortality rates. If all countries had the Japanese rates, the lowest in the world, there would be only one-million child deaths each year, instead of the current eleven million deaths. Seven out of ten deaths in children under the age of five years still occur in low-income countries and can be attributed to just five preventable conditions—pneumonia, diarrhoeal diseases, malaria, measles, and malnutrition; these conditions overlap and are exacerbated by poverty. Although the eradication of polio is likely to be completed in the near future, the goal of vaccinating 90 percent of children under five years against measles by 2000 has not been reached. Indeed, global coverage declined from 79 percent in 1997 to 72 percent in 1998 [46].

Maternal mortality data are equally distressing, even though maternal deaths make up only about 1 percent of all deaths. Although maternal deaths are often hard to measure and classify accurately, the maternal mortality rates vary enormously from as low as six per 100,000 in Australia to 1800 per 100,000 in Sierra Leone.

The fragility of health gains

The fragility of recent health gains has become apparent in the face of social disruption as a result of economic and political disarray, as in the former Soviet Union (see Chapter 5), or civil war, as in the former Yugoslavia. Less spectacular, but equally disturbing, is the recent increase in young adult male mortality in several northern and southern European countries. While the final pathway appears to be through alcohol in the north, HIV/AIDS and traffic crashes are responsible in the south [47].

Around thirty-seven million people worldwide are currently living with HIV/AIDS, and 95 percent of them are in developing countries. In many countries, the development gains of the past fifty years, including the increase in child survival and in life expectancy are being wiped out by the HIV/AIDS epidemic. In Zimbabwe, for example, life expectancy at birth for men is expected to fall from the present fifty-two years to forty-one years by 2005. In the absence of AIDS it would have been expected to rise to sixty-six years by 2005 [48]. In Tanzania and other parts of Africa, infant mortality is on the increase in part due to the collapse of the public health system. In sub-Saharan Africa, where nearly twenty-five million people are infected, HIV/AIDS is now the leading cause of death with more women being infected than men. HIV infection is also increasing rapidly in Asia, particularly in south and south-east Asia, with six million people currently infected. A special UN Security Council meeting on HIV/AIDS crisis in Africa referred to it as a unique modern-day plague that threatens the political, economic and social stability of sub-Saharan Africa and Asia [49].

Old and new public health challenges

The main item on the development agenda is the over one billion people whose life experiences have improved only slowly over the last half-century. Almost two-thirds of poor people live in Asia and the Pacific region with 17 percent in Africa and 10 percent in the rest of the world; a substantial majority of the poor are women. The excluded billion need to be placed more firmly on the international development agenda, and increasingly this is being addressed through health programmes as well as more directly by economic means. A major goal of this agenda is the reduction by half of the number of people living in absolute poverty by the year 2015. Opinions differ as to whether this goal is achievable. Officially, the WHO is optimistic that, with a collaborative effort, this goal is attainable. However, progress is slow and while the proportion of people living in extreme poverty fell in the last decade, the actual number of people living in poverty increased in South Asia and sub-Saharan Africa owing to the failure of current policies of economic growth. Many national anti-poverty action plans remain vague and limited by poor governance and do not consider the multidimensional nature of poverty [50].

A feature of the current global health status picture is the "double burden" of disease. Countries that are still struggling with old and new infectious disease epidemics must now also deal with the emerging epidemics of chronic noncommunicable disease such as heart disease, stroke, diabetes and cancer. Already just five risk factors—unsafe sexual practices, alcohol use, indoor air pollution, occupational exposures and tobacco use account for at least 20 percent of the world's disease burden. Tobacco use continues to increase in developing countries suggesting that the global impact on disease will also increase. Current estimates suggest that there were 4.8 million preventable tobacco caused deaths; in 2000; estimates for the year 2020 suggest that this number will increase to 9 million. More than three quarters of these deaths are due to just three causes: cardiovascular disease, lung cancer, and chronic respiratory disease.

The noncommunicable disease burden becomes especially evident as populations age and as population risk factor profiles change, partly in response to global pressures. In the developed countries the ageing of the population is occurring in a relatively slow and predictable manner, and in some, such as Japan and Sweden, the rate of ageing is already slowing down. Already more than half (57 percent) of the world's population over the age of sixty-five years lives in developing countries. The proportion of the world's population over sixty-five years, currently 7 percent, will more than double (to 16 percent) in the next fifty years. The most explosive ageing will occur in some of the poorer regions of the world, particularly in India, Indonesia, and China; within the next half century, the number of people aged sixty-five years or more will increase six-fold in the South East Asian region of the WHO [48].

These rapid demographic changes, particularly in poorer regions of the world, will lead to an increase in the burden of noncommunicable diseases in the absence of preventive action. The noncommunicable disease epidemics are essentially preventable according to existing knowledge. Over the last fifty years an extensive body of research has accumulated in different settings using a variety of methods including laboratory, clinical methods, and quantitative and qualitative population sciences. It is well known, for example, that the major established risk factors common to many noncommunicable diseases (smoking, high blood pressure, inadequate diet, lack of physical activity), are responsible for most of the occurrence of premature cardiovascular disease in developed countries [51,52]. This research has identified appropriate strategies for the prevention and control of noncommunicable disease and some of these lessons have been applied with good effect in wealthy countries. Efforts to reduce population cardiovascular disease risk factor levels, for example, have contributed to an important decline in cardiovascular disease death rates in many developed countries [53,54] and tobacco-attributable mortality is now declining among men in several of these countries.

The causes of the noncommunicable disease epidemics in developing countries appear to be largely the same as in wealthy countries [55]. The challenge will be to translate this knowledge into effective action in developing countries in order to avoid the predictable, but largely preventable, burden of noncommunicable diseases. It is difficult for poorer countries to focus on medium-term preventive strategies in the face of more immediate health problems, even though over 40 percent of all deaths in the poorest 20 percent of the world's population are already due to noncommunicable diseases. The "double burden" of disease is being superceded by the "triple burden". To the unfinished agendas of infectious and noncommunicable disease prevention and control, is being added new health threats consequent on the new phase of globalization (see Chapter 1). These new challenges will potentially worsen regional and national health inequalities [56].

Conclusions

Improvements in global health status as measured by gains in life expectancy and other measures and the reductions in preventable deaths, have been accompanied by a widening health and poverty gap between and within countries. Investment in health research and development remains focused largely on the health problems of the 10 percent of the world's richest populations and only 10 percent of funds available for health research is directed at improving the health of 90 percent of the world's population. This disparity, referred to as the 10/90 disequilibrium [57], requires urgent attention.

People living in poor countries not only face lower life expectancies than those in richer countries but also live a higher proportion of their lives in poor health. Richer countries should be much more active in seeking ways to improve the health of the world's poor. The WHO has been a strong advocate for efforts to increase the resources available for this purpose. The recent WHO Commission on Macroeconomics and Health took an optimistic view of the relationship between health expenditure/interventions and health outcomes. It concluded that the bulk of the global disease burden is the result of a relatively small set of conditions, each with an existing set of effective interventions [58]. The main problems are the funding of these interventions and access of poor populations to these interventions. The Commission estimated that the essential interventions to target these problems could be provided for a per capita cost of around $34 per person per year or a total annual increase in health expenditures of around $17 billion by 2007 and $29 billion by 2015, above the level of 2002.

Routine health status measures of health trends and inequalities are required to heighten awareness of their significance among policy makers, donors and international agencies. Better and more comprehensive data is a first step in the development of a stronger strategy to improve overall health and reduce inequalities in health status throughout the world. There is insufficient emphasis given to disease surveillance in most national health systems, a serious impediment to setting disease prevention and control priorities and for measuring progress. Additionally, there is as yet insufficient emphasis in national health data collection systems on the need for cross-population comparability. Despite the growing pressures of shrinking public sector resources, there is an urgent need for centralized organizations to collect data [59]. There is a danger of this process becoming increasingly fragmented as a result of growing reliance upon private and voluntary sector organizations to collect such data.

The global health scene has been characterised by major steps forward but with some disturbing features. The measurement of health status is multi-faceted and must take account of differences between and within nations that inevitably impinge on the comparability of data. As a first and essential step there is need for better national and regional heath surveillance systems [60]. Without such data, particularly in poorer regions of the world, it will be difficult to know if, and how much, progress is being made in improving global health status and reducing growing health inequalities.

Acknowledgments

The authors thank WHO staff and others who have contributed to the measurement of global health status, in particular Omar Ahmad, Jose Ayuso, Somnath Chatterji, Mie Inoue, Matilde Leonardi, Alan Lopez, Rafael Lozano, Doris Ma Fat, Brodie Ferguson, Chris Murray, Ritu Sadana, Joshua Salomon, Claudia Stein and Bedirhan Ustun.

References

[1] Lopez AD, Murray CJL, Ahmad O et al. *Life Tables for 191 Countries for 2000*. Geneva: WHO, 2002.

[2] Lopez AD. Counting the dead in China: Measuring tobacco's impact in developing world. *BMJ* 1998; 317: 1399–400.

[3] Office of the Registrar General, Government of India, New Delhi, India (personal Communication).

[4] Chandramohan D, Maude G, Rodrigues LC, Hayes RJ. Verbal Autopsies for adult deaths: Issues in their development and validation. *Int J Epidemiol* 1994; 23: 313–22.

[5] Hoj C, Stensballe J, Aabz P. Maternal mortality in Guinea Bisseau: the use of verbal autopsies in a multi ethnic population. *Int J Epidemiol* 1999; 28: 70–6.

[6] Morris L, Danel I, Stupp P, Sarbanescu F. Household surveys to evaluate reproductive health programmes. In M. Khlat (ed.). *Demographic Evaluation of Health Programmes*. UNFPA, French Ministry of Cooperation. 1996; pp. 75–87.

[7] Murray CJM, King G, Lopez A et al. Armed conflict as a public health problem. *BMJ* 2002; **324**: 346–9.

[8] World Health Organization. World Health Report 2000. Health Systems: Improving Performance. Geneva: WHO, 2000.

[9] World Health Organization. World Health Report 2001. Mental health: New Understanding, New Hope. Geneva: WHO, 2001.

[10] Salomon JA, Murray CJL. Modelling HIV/AIDS epidemics in sub-Saharan Africa using seroprevalence data from antenatal clinics. *Bull WHO* 2001; **79**: 596–607.

[11] McDowell I, Newell C. *Measuring Health: a Guide to Rating Scales and Questionnaires*, 2nd edn. New York: Oxford University Press, 1996.

[12] World Health Organization. International Classification of Impairments, Disabilities, and Handicaps. Geneva: WHO, 1980 (Reprint 1993).

[13] World Health Organization. ICF: International classification of functioning, disability and health. Geneva: WHO, 2001.

[14] Johansson SR. The health transition: the cultural inflation of morbidity during the decline of mortality. *Health Transition Review* 1991; **1**: 39–68.

[15] Sadana R, Mathers CD, Lopez A et al. Comparative analysis of more than 50 household surveys of health status. In: CJL Murray, JA Salomon, CD Mathers, AD Lopez (eds.). *Summary Measures of Population Health: Concepts, Ethics, Measurement and Applications*. Geneva: WHO, 2002.

[16] Üstün TB, Chatterji S, Villanueva M et al. WHO Multi-country Household Survey Study on Health and Responsiveness, 2000–2001. GPE discussion paper No. 37. Geneva: WHO, 2001.

[17] Murray CJL, Tandon A, Salomon J, Mathers CD. New approaches to enhance cross-population comparability of survey results. In: CJL Murray, JA Salomon, CD Mathers, AD Lopez (eds.). *Summary Measures of Population Health: Concepts, Ethics, Measurement and Applications*. Geneva: WHO, 2002.

[18] Murray CJL, Salomon JA, Mathers CD. A critical examination of summary measures of population health. *Bull WHO* 2000; **78**: 981–94.

[19] Murray CJL, Lopez AD (eds.). The global burden of disease: a comprehensive assessment of mortality and disability from diseases, injuries and risk factors in 1990 and projected to 2020. *Global Burden of disease and Injury Series*, Vol. 1. Cambridge: Harvard University Press, 1996.

[20] Lai D, Hardy RJ. Potential gains in life expectancy or years of potential life lost: Impact of competing risks of death. *Int J Epidemiol* 1999; **28**: 894–8.

[21] Mathers CD, Vos T, Lopez AD, Ezzati M. *National Burden of Disease Studies: A Practical Guide. Edition 2.0*. Geneva: WHO, 2001.

[22] Sayers B McA, Bailey NTJ et al. The disability adjusted life year concept: A comment. European *J Pub Hlth* 1997; 7: 113.

[23] Williams A. Calculating the global burden of disease: time for a strategic reappraisal? *Health Econ* 1998; 8: 1–8.

[24] Murray CJL, Lopez AD. Progress and directions in refining the global burden of disease approach: response to Williams. *Health Econ* 2000; 9: 69–82.

[25] Cooper RS, Osotimehin B, Kaufman JS, Forrester T. Disease burden in sub-Saharan Africa: what should we conclude in the absence of data? *Lancet* 1998; 351: 208–10.

[26] Barendregt JJ, Bonneux L, Vander Maas PJ. DALYs: the age-weight on balance. *Bull WHO* 1996; 74: 439–43.

[27] Barker C, Green A. Opening the debate on DALYs. *Hlth Pol Planning* 1996; 11: 179–83.

[28] Mathers C, Vos T, Stevenson C. The burden of disease and injury in Australia. Canberra: Australian Institute of Health and Welfare, 1999.

[29] Editorial. The World Bank's cure for donor fatigue. *Lancet* 1993; 342: 63–4.

[30] Gwatkin DR, Guillot M, Heuveline P. The burden of disease among the global poor. *Lancet* 1999; 354: 586–89.

[31] Gwatkin DR, Guillot M. *The Burden of Disease Among the Global Poor: Current Situation, Future Trends, and Implications for Strategy*. Washington, DC: The World Bank, 2000.

[32] Robine JM, Romieu I, Cambois E. Health expectancy indicators. *Bull WHO* 1999; 77: 181–5.

[33] OECD. Eco-santé (OECD Health Database). Paris: OECD, 1999.

[34] Robine JM, Mathers CD, Brouard N. Trends and differentials in disability-free life expectancy: Concepts, methods and findings. In: G. Caselli, A Lopez (ed.). *Health and Mortality Among Elderly Populations*. Oxford: Clarendon Press, 1996, pp. 182–201.

[35] Mathers CD, Sadana R, Salomon J et al. Healthy life expectancy in 191 countries, 1999. *Lancet* 2001; 357: 1685–91.

[36] Almeida C, Braveman P, Gold MR et al. Methodological concerns and recommendations on policy consequences of the World Health Report 2000. *Lancet* 2001; 357: 1692–97.

[37] Sadana R, Tandon A, Serdobova I et al. Describing population health in six domains: comparable results from 66 household surveys. Global Program on Evidence for Health policy Discussion Paper No. 43, Geneva: WHO, 2002.

[38] Mathers CD, Murray CJL, Lopez AD et al. Estimates of healthy life expectancy for 191 countries in the year 2000: methods and results (GPE discussion paper No. 38). Geneva: WHO, 2001.

[39] Shkolnikov V, McKee M, Leon, D. Changes in life expectancy in Russia in the mid-1990s. *Lancet* 2001; 357: 917–21.

[40] Gavrilova NS, Semyonova VG, Evdokushkina GN, Gavrilov LA. The response of violent mortality to economic crisis in Russia. *Population Research and Policy Review* 2000; **19**: 397–419.

[41] Chakravorty L. Biological Stress and History from below: Millet zone of India 1970–1992. In: I Qadeer, K Sen, KR Nayar (eds.). *Public Health and the Poverty of Reforms in South Asia at the Turn of the Century*. Sage: New Delhi, 2000.

[42] Murray CJL, Michaud CM, McKenna MT, Marks JS. *US patterns of mortality by county and race: 1965–1994*. National Centre for Chronic Disease Prevention and Health Promotion, Atlanta and Harvard Centre for Population and Development Studies, Cambridge, USA.

[43] Tüchsen F, Endahl LA. Increasing inequality in ischaemic heart disease among employed men in Denmark 1981–1993: the need for a new preventive policy. *Int J Epidemiol* 1999; **28**: 640–4.

[44] Drever F, Whitehead M. Health Inequalities: Decennial Supplement. London: The Stationery Office, 1997.

[45] Wnuk-Lipinski E, Illsley R. International comparative analysis: main findings and conclusions. *Soc Sci Med* 1990; **31**: 879–89.

[46] Editorial. Measles, MMR, and autism: the confusion continues. *Lancet* 2000; **355**: 1379.

[47] Leon DA, Chenet L, Shkolnikov VM et al. Huge variation in Russian mortality rates 1984–1994: artefact, alcohol, or what? *Lancet* 1997; **350**: 383–8.

[48] United Nations. Revision of the World Population Estimates and Projections. 1998.

[49] Brundtland GH. We have rekindled a spirit of global solidarity. Press release. 53rd World Health Assembly, 20 May 2000.

[50] Overcoming Human Poverty. Poverty Report 2000. United Nations Development Programme. New York: New York, 2000.

[51] Magnus P, Beaglehole R. Real contribution of the major risk factors to the coronary epidemics. Time to end the "only 50% myth". *Arch Intern Med* 2001; **161**: 2657–60.

[52] Stamler J, Stamler R, Neaton JD et al. Low risk-factor profile and long term cardiovascular and non-cardiovascular mortality and life expectancy. Findings for 5 large cohorts of young adult and middle-aged men and women. *JAMA* 1999; **282**: 2012–18.

[53] Kuulasmaa K, Tunstall-Pedoe H, Dobson A et al. For the WHO MONICA Project. Estimation of contribution of changes in classic risk factors to trends in coronary-event rates across the WHO MONICA Project populations. *Lancet* 2000; **355**: 675–87.

[54] Vartiainen E, Jousilahti P, Alftahan G et al. Cardiovascular risk factor changes in Finland, 1972–1997. *Int J Epidemiol* 2000; **29**: 49–56.

[55] Eastern Stroke and Coronary Heart Disease Collaborative Research Group. Blood pressure, cholesterol, and stroke in eastern Asia. *Lancet* 1998; **352**: 1801–7.

[56] McMichael AJ, Beaglehole R. The changing global context of public health. *Lancet* 2000; **356**: 495–99.

[57] Global Forum for Health Research. The 10/90 Report on Health Research 2000. Geneva: Global Forum for Health Research, 2001.

[58] Commission on Macroeconomics and Health. Macroeconomics and health: Investing in Health for Economic Development. Geneva: WHO, 2001.

[59] Qadeer I, Sen K. Public health debacle in South Asia: a reflection of the crisis in welfarism: *J Pub Hlth Med* 1998; **20**: 93–6.

[60] Bonita R, Winkelmann R, Douglas K, de Courten M. The WHO stepwise approach to surveillance (STEPS) of non-communicable disease risk factors. In: McQueen DV and Puska P (editors), *Global Risk Factor Surveillance.* London: Kluwer Academic/Plenum Publishers, in press.

Chapter 3

Public health in the United Kingdom

Sian Griffiths

This chapter identifies the main public health challenges in the United Kingdom, with a focus on England, and critically analyses the recent developments in health policy, the organizational changes in the National Health Service in 2002 and their impact on public health practice in the United Kingdom.

Background

Public health has been a function of the National Health Service (NHS) since 1974. Before this time it was the responsibility of local government with each local council having a medical officer of health (MoH) responsible for the health of the population. The MoH's job was to advise the council, in particular through the production of an annual report detailing communicable disease outbreaks and control measures, as well as describing issues within the domains of social care, environmental health and community health services. The changes in the 1970s brought together in the NHS the three strands of modern public health—health protection, medical management and preventive health services—as reflected in the most widely used definition:

> The science and art of preventing disease, prolonging life and promoting health through the organised efforts of society [1].

The changes also created independent environmental health and social work professions. Since that time the frequent changes within the structure and organization of the NHS have influenced the way public health professionals work within the health service and with other agencies such as local government. These changes have not always been to the advantage of public health professionals. In 2002 change is once more on the agenda with the threat of recurrent upheaval. There are also opportunities for public health to reduce health inequalities and create new ways of working, not only within the NHS but also within communities in partnership with local government and local people.

The challenge of inequalities

One of the biggest challenges for public health is to address the health inequalities which continue to grow. People are living longer in the United Kingdom, but the increased length of life is unevenly distributed between social groups and the extra years are not necessarily healthy years. There has been a consistent widening of the health gap between social classes [2]. The most recent decennial supplement on health inequalities showed that whilst mortality has decreased overall, the greatest decreases have occurred in the most advantaged groups (social class "one") [3]. During the period 1972–1996 the life expectancy for men in social class one was 77.7 years, a gap of nine years between them and social class five for whom life expectancy was 68.2 years. These figures reflect a differential increase over this period for social class one men of an additional 5.7 years compared with 1.7 years for those in social class five.

Not only are there social class differences in life expectancy, but there are also geographical differences; men in England can expect to live 2.6 years longer than their Scottish counterparts, and Scottish women 2.1 years less than their English neighbors. The differential between better health in the south of England than in the north is a consistent finding in studies on coronary heart disease and associated health behaviors [2]. Health behaviors also show marked differences by social class. The health survey for England [4] found that 15 percent of social class one men were smokers compared with 42 percent of those in social class five; 7 percent of social class one women had a high fat diet compared with 17 percent of social class five women; in men the figures were 19 percent and 38 percent respectively.

These figures demonstrate higher levels of behaviors risky for health amongst the most socially disadvantaged. Some other groups also remain at particular disadvantage. Death rates from coronary heart disease among first generation south Asians aged 20–69 are about 50 percent higher than the England and Wales average. The death rate for stroke among people aged 20–69 born in the Caribbean is more than 50 percent greater than the England and Wales average. Perinatal mortality among Pakistani born mothers is nearly twice the United Kingdom average. Diagnoses of schizophrenia are 3–6 times higher among the African–Caribbean groups than in the white population [2]. These data highlight one of the major challenges facing public health professionals in the United Kingdom which are underlined further when compared with Europe. Not only is the health budget in the United Kingdom amongst the lowest in terms of percentage of GDP, but health outcomes such as mortality rates for common cancers are also worse in the United Kingdom [5].

Developments in health policy

The election of a Labour government in 1997 heralded a major shift in health policy for the United Kingdom. The NHS Plan [7] produced by the new government in 2000 outlined the move away from the purchaser/provider split of the internal market towards a whole systems approach. This model is typified by a greater focus on patient involvement and choice, an emphasis on development of intermediate care and changes to patterns of acute care with greater freedom at a local level. In particular, the reorganization gives clinicians and primary care organizations the levers to drive improvement in health as well as delivery of health care.

Greater awareness of the impact of the wider determinants on health and a government wide commitment to reducing inequalities were reflected in the creation of a Minister for Public Health and in Saving Lives—Our Healthier Nation (OHN) [6], the government's public health strategy published in 1999. OHN and the proposals within it were heralded as a new, modern approach to public health. The prime minister highlighted three complementary strands of action to improve health: individuals and their families taking action for themselves; the help which could be offered by communities working together in partnership; and the key role of government in addressing the major determinants of health such as housing, jobs and education as summarized in Box 3.1.

Although the strategy was welcomed warmly by public health professionals, its objectives and implementation have been overshadowed by the acute care agenda of the NHS Plan [7]. Many of the initiatives within Saving Lives are still under development. For example, the Healthy Living Centers programme funded by lottery monies has yet to complete its financial allocations. Healthy Living Centers (HLCs) are, like Health Action Zones, a good example of the reawakening of the interest in civic society and community engagement in health. Their objective is to target deprived communities and, through engaging the local community with statutory agencies, provide opportunities to link sectors to offer local people opportunities to improve their health. Successful bids

Box 3.1 Key elements of Saving Lives—Our Healthier Nation

- a focus on reducing inequalities in health;
- promoting awareness of the wider determinants of health;
- the need for health impact assessment and establishment of observatories to monitor health;
- setting targets for the major killers of cancer, coronary heart disease, stroke, accidents, mental health;
- identifying the need for wider action;
- developing partnerships through primary care, health improvement programmes, healthy living centres, health action zones;
- setting standards and developing the specialist and practitioner workforce; and
- establishment of the Health Development Agency to support public health development.

have included a wide variety of initiatives some of which are capital based building projects; others are for revenue for staff and local activities to promote health.

The HLC programme has funded both local and national initiatives. One example of a national initiative is the Walking the Way to Health programme, a national scheme in partnership with the British Heart Foundation, the Countryside Agency and the private sector [8]. Evaluation of the pilot study on which the bid was based demonstrated the health gains from a programme which promotes walking both as a social and a healthy activity for all ages [9]. By extending the scheme to areas of deprivation it is hoped to have an environmental and social impact as well as contributing to health goals such as improved heart health, a reduction in problems associated with obesity, and improved balance, flexibility and co-ordination amongst the older participating population. The impact of the project will be fully evaluated. The short term nature of this and other projects does, however, undermine the opportunities for assessing longer term impacts. There is increasing pressure on all government departments to make projects sustainable, provided initial evaluation demonstrates progress [10].

The Health Development Agency, which replaced the Health Education Authority, is playing a key role in assimilating evidence on effective preventive and community interventions. It is also disseminating information to and between community based projects as well as supporting evidence based interventions as part of national service frameworks. The National Electronic Library for Health, part of a government e-learning initiative to make best use of IT and manage knowledge, will also assist dissemination of evidence.

The absence of research evidence to demonstrate the effectiveness of community projects remains a challenge and weakens the bid for greater investment in public health programmes. The lack of evidence on the effectiveness of the components of multifaceted interventions such as HLCs, highlights the relative lack of research into community based initiatives.

Community based developments which improve health are now formally recognized as integral to the NHS; a greater awareness has been created within the health service of their importance and the need for public health skills at local level to initiate, co-ordinate and evaluate them. Identifying and protecting resources for public health activity remains a challenge because of competition with the illness service provided by the NHS which takes priority.

Policy development

The public health agenda set out in Saving Lives [6] has led to a variety of policy initiatives. The Acheson report [1] reviewed evidence of effective action to combat health inequalities and emphasized the relatively small contribution of the health service to the reduction of inequalities. The broader social inclusion agenda has also been developed and championed through the work of the social exclusion unit [11]. Increasingly there is awareness of potential impact on health of government policies from other departments. For example, the Chancellor of the Exchequer is committed to eradicating child poverty through policies such as Family Tax Credit and by the emphasis given to children within all areas of social policy, not just those concerned with education or child health. High profile initiatives such as Surestart [12] which bridge sectors demonstrate this commitment. Other examples include: identifying the health benefits of the National Cycling Strategy [13]; the work of youth offending teams [14]; and the consideration of the health impacts of agricultural and farming policies. The case for putting health into the heart of public policy has been made in a recent report on food and farming [15]. This report highlights the need to identify links between health and production and consumption, taking into account sustainability, trade liberalization, food safety, access and other issues.

However, one of the problems in identifying this broad type of activity as central to the work of public health has been that, welcome as these reports are, gaining public profile and support remain difficult. For historic reasons the official focus on public health in the United Kingdom continues to sit within the NHS, exemplified by the position within the Department of Health in England of the Minister for Public Health [16]. This positioning is problematic because of the continual over emphasis in the media and by ministers on acute health services, resulting in a relatively low profile for public health issues. The health gain from promoting better health and preventing disease may well be more cost effective as demonstrated by QALY analysis for interventions in coronary heart disease and cancer [17]. However, the focus remains largely on the government's need to meet targets for operations and waiting lists.

This priority is exemplified by the NHS Plan published in July 2000 [7]. The Plan was primarily focused on service delivery, particularly on meeting election pledges around waiting lists and times, and training more doctors and nurses. Within the plan, the objectives of Saving Lives [6] are reflected through commitment to National Service Frameworks (NSFs) for major diseases (cancer, heart disease, diabetes) as well as recognition of the importance of addressing the wider determinants of health and decreasing health inequalities. The structural changes proposed promote public health with the creation of primary care organizations and with the adoption of public health perspectives and principles within other central initiatives. However, the overall focus remains on the acute sector.

National health service frameworks and public health

The policy links between Saving Lives [6] and the Plan [7] are made through the care pathway approach to tackling major health programmes for cancer, heart disease, mental health, diabetes, older people and children. The care pathway approach follows the pathway from health promotion/disease prevention through treatment and rehabilitation to long term care. This approach to disease management moves public health initiatives into the mainstream delivery of the NHS (see Box 3.2).

Box 3.2   Examples of public health activity in coronary heart disease care pathway

Health promotion: support free fruit to schools; evaluation of local smoking cessation programme.

Prevention: audit of measurement of hypertension by GPs in primary care.

Acute care: service planning, including workforce needed, to meet targets for coronary artery bypass grafting.

Rehabilitation: input to cardiac rehabilitation programmes run jointly with local authorities.

Long term follow up: work with local voluntary sector to provide support at home for stroke patient.

For each stage of the process there is the requirement to consider how inequalities in health are being addressed.

Inequalities

Addressing inequalities was a key theme within OHN [6]. More recently a consultation was held on the formal adoption of targets for inequalities [18]. The proposed targets were: starting with children under one year, by 2010 to reduce by at least 10 percent the gap in mortality between manual groups and the population as a whole; and starting with health authorities, by 2010 to reduce by at least 10 percent the gap between the fifth of areas with the lowest life expectancy at birth and the population as a whole [18].

The key messages from the consultation reiterated that the health service alone could not address inequalities and sustainable public policy was needed at local level to link the themes and targets across the broader public health remit. There was general agreement with what needed to be done, but concern at the low priority within the NHS, despite the rhetoric of commitment. The other major anxiety was the current reorganization and the fragility of the new structures—Local Strategic Partnerships and Primary Care Organizations—which would be expected to deliver at a local level.

One of the elements of this fragility is funding for public health initiatives. The relevance of addressing inequalities as part of future funding of the NHS has been considered as part of a cross cutting review by the Treasury in its Comprehensive Spending Review (CSR) which will influence future national financial strategies. Part of the CSR process, the Wanless report [19], begins "*Ill health in adulthood is associated with poverty*".

Further reference is made to the impact of broader determinants of health, for example, economic, environmental and lifestyle factors. Most importantly, the need to increase healthy life expectancy is identified and also the need to change levels of morbidity by tackling smoking, poverty and inequality, diet, exercise, alcohol and pollution. To quote: "*Tackling poverty or pollution or reducing smoking will require action beyond the health service . . . other parts of government or society have more scope to influence these factors than the NHS. This raises the question of how much of any additional resources should be spent on health care and in particular on the NHS*".[19] The Wanless report postulated three scenarios—slow progress with no change in momentum, solid progress with NHS service improvements, and a fully engaged scenario in which the health service is responsive with high rates of technology uptake, particularly in relation to disease prevention. The modeling suggests that such a fully engaged scenario, in which prevention and public engagement in health are high on the agenda, will be the most effective in terms of costs as well as health outcomes.

The longer term benefits of investing in prevention programmes, with their lower political appeal and less obvious and less well researched impacts, are again overshadowed by the shorter term imperatives of possible gains from more doctors and quicker throughputs. Even within the choice of subjects to pick for evaluation by the National Institute for Clinical Excellence (NICE), there is a bias towards drugs which will show results in acute conditions.

The challenge facing public health is to demonstrate its relevance within this acute care-focused policy context. The Select Committee in 2000 [16] into public health struggled with definitions. Their deliberations demonstrated that there is confusion about the phrase public health at all levels. To appeal to those allocating resources as well as those unfamiliar with population based health approaches, public health goals need to be clearly and concretely expressed. This can be achieved by constructing a public health service with public health programmes and setting targets which enable these programmes to be "performance managed" for their delivery of explicit processes and health improvement. For example, a programme on smoking cessation should demonstrate how many smokers have attended clinics, how many received counselling and prescriptions and how many quit smoking. Over time there should be a demonstrable decrease in mortality contributing to meeting the targets set for reductions in heart disease and cancer. Such an approach fits within the NHS Plan [7] by integrating into both the care pathways of the NSF and into the specific proposals for reducing inequalities. The proposals for reducing inequalities include: the establishment of targets by government, ensuring children have a healthy start in life, delivering programmes to promote healthy diets and lifestyles, and creating new partnerships with local government.

Approaching public health within this framework can be criticized as a reductionist approach which adopts a biomedical model. However, without this clarity there is a risk of much public health talk but little public health action and no commitment of resources. Public health could be everyone's business and no ones responsibility, leading to a belief system with no delivery mechanism.

Organization of public health practice in the United Kingdom

To add to this policy challenge, the current modernization process of the NHS [7] has created the largest set of organizational changes faced by the public health service in the United Kingdom since 1974. Public health is being redefined within the emerging new organizational structures for the NHS within each of the four countries within the United Kingdom. The context for the changes in public health were set in 2001 by the Select Committee (SC) report on the future of public health [16], the report on the public health function by the Chief Medical Officer of England [24] and the political speech from the Secretary of State for Health [20] which announced the structural changes later developed in Shifting the Balance of Power [22].

Select committee

The SC public health review assessed the current public health function and its co-ordination and studied alternative models for provision. Alan Millburn, Secretary of State, told the committee: *the time has come to take public health out of the ghetto* [20] reinforcing the renewed commitment by government to health as well as health services. The main areas for recommendations from the committee are shown in Box 3.3.

The Chief Medical Officer's report on the Public Health Function [24]

Six major themes were identified by the Chief Medical Officer (CMO) as important (Box 3.4). One of the major areas within the report is the need to develop and strengthen the multidisciplinary nature of the public health workforce: *specialists working in the NHS in future may come from a variety of professional backgrounds... They will have a common core of knowledge, skills and experience acquired from post graduate public health qualifications and successful completion of approved training, and experience gained in practice* [24]. Movement in this direction has been made very much easier by the

Faculty of Public Health Medicine, the relevant specialist professional body, agreeing to widen its membership from a solely medical base and to accept specialists on the basis of meeting equivalent standards through training and examinations. These standards exist for ten key areas of public health practice, see Box 3.5.

These have been accepted as the basis for training, continuing professional development, appraisal and revalidation of public health specialists (further detail is on the Faculty web site. *www.fphm.org.uk*).

Box 3.3 The key themes from the Select Committee review of Public Health [16]

- the need to achieve balance in health policy between health and health care, and between upstream and downstream policies;
- strengthening public health leadership at all levels;
- establishing strong partnerships at all levels for a broad based approach to public health;
- placing the emphasis on public health practice and implementation rather than on knowledge acquisition for its own sake;
- creating incentives for health improvement;
- building the evidence base in public health;
- learning the lessons from past failures or partial successes in putting health before health care.

Box 3.4 Themes from CMO's report

There needs to be:
- a wider understanding of health and well being;
- better co-ordination and communication within the public health function;
- effective 'joined up working', particularly with local government;
- sustained community development and public involvement;
- an increase in capacity and capabilities in the public health function;
- development of public health practice, health protection, primary care and acute care trusts.

Box 3.5 Key areas for specialist public health practice [21]

1. *Surveillance and assessment of the population's health* and well-being (including managing, analyzing and interpreting information, knowledge and statistics).
2. *Promoting and protecting the population's health* and well-being.
3. Developing *quality and risk management* within an evaluative culture.
4. *Collaborative* working for health.
5. Developing *health programmes and services and reducing inequalities*.
6. *Policy and strategy* development and implementation.
7. Working with and for *communities*.
8. *Strategic leadership* for health.
9. *Research and development*.
10. *Ethically* managing self, people and resources (including education and continuing professional development).

Shifting the Balance of Power [22]

Each of the four countries within the UK felt organizational change. The current changes in the English public health service are the unintended consequence of structural changes announced in April 2001 in a pre election speech by the Secretary of State [20]. These changes have a major impact on public health professionals and the future delivery of the public health function. Shifting the Balance of Power [22] emphasizes the key themes of devolution of decision making to front line clinicians and local people. The creation of primary care based organizations which organize local care, commission from hospitals and work with local authorities on improving health, has promoted a major change in public health organizations. *These organizational changes have provided the opportunity to review the way significant functions are delivered across the NHS with new more appropriate arrangements for public health . . . .*[22] Organizationally there will be a strong public health team in every Primary Care Trust (PCT) focused on improving health, preventing serious illness and reducing inequalities in the populations served. There will be a Director of Public Health (DPH) in every PCT with clear links into newly created public health networks with skills, knowledge and experience in every area designed according to local needs and circumstances.

PCTs will need a range of skills and appropriately trained staff to deliver their new responsibilities. For example, all the workforce will need to focus on public health interventions with public health practitioners delivering specific programmes. Public health specialists will assess health needs, develop effective strategies in partnership with relevant agencies, and monitor progress towards achieving outcomes, particularly reductions of health inequalities. The style of public health leadership will be expected to shift from the previous "remote" style, inherent with working for health authorities, to a style which fits the following description: *She or he will be well known, respected and credible with local people—particularly those in the most deprived communities, local authorities, general practitioners and other local clinicians. They will be accessible to the local media, explaining and educating on health and inequalities issues . . . they will have a team whose composition is a local matter for determination . . . they will also seek to ensure that the public health role of the primary care workforce [e.g., health visitors, school nurses, health promotion, other community workers] is fully realized by encouraging practitioners to lead specific programmes.*[22]

With the focus on improving health, there is an expectation that the boundaries will increasingly be blurred between local government and the NHS. The Select Committee [16] debated the possible relocation of public health in local government but finally agreed that the most effective way of delivering the public health service was to agree locally the best way of bringing partners together. There are opportunities for developing new models of delivery such as joint appointments of DPHs between NHS and local councils, pooled resources to create joint units, and local authority membership of public health teams, which will work to deliver the new Local Strategic Partnerships (LSPs). The LSPs are required of local government and are the new agreements which will examine how local authorities are delivering all their services, including their responsibility for the social, environmental and economic factors which impact on health. In his speech laying out the future for public health, the minister emphasized the key role of LSPs and community plans in both raising the profile of the public health role of local government and the need to *ensure that engagement in the public health agenda is equally achieved in local government work . . . we expect that the links between public health and environmental health to be further strengthened and enhanced* [23].

The developing health protection agenda

Saving Lives [6] committed government to reviewing the existing services for communicable disease control. The cumulative effect of the re-emergence of TB, emergence of new infections such as CJD, increased global travel and the threats of bioterrorism, raised the profile not only of the control of infectious disease but also the need for links to chemical risks to health [24]. The events of 11 September 2001 in the United States highlighted the need for a co-ordinated and rapid response to the threats of bioterrorism including a capacity to plan for such emergencies. In Getting Ahead of the Curve [25], the CMO for England has offered a blueprint for a new agency, the National Infection Control and Health Protection Agency, which will, by combining existing bodies, enable improved co-ordination and surveillance and detection of disease as well as rapid response to threats and epidemics.

Networks

Networking is a core theme running through the modernization process. For public health, networks will be critical for maintaining skills and expertise, for allowing responsiveness at appropriate population levels, and for ensuring training and continuing professional development. The definition of a public health network is: *Linked groups of public health professionals working in a co-ordinated manner across organizations and structural boundaries who will have a common agenda to promote health and reduce health inequalities for given populations* [26]. Networks will be needed at different population levels. For example, an electronic network at national level to share existing skills and knowledge is proposed. Public Health Observatories, another innovation within the OHN strategy, will contribute at the regional level by providing information on health, health determinants and health service responses. Networks will enable sharing of scarce public health skills, including those in universities, and support public health governance. However, to reach their potential the task of defining, managing and developing these networks must be addressed.

Public Health in other settings

The focus of change has been the organizational structures around regions and primary care. There will still be a developing role for public health approaches and expertise within the acute hospital sector. Public health specialists are increasingly playing a role in improving quality of care and working closely with clinical colleagues to implement evidence based care.

The new arrangements also create opportunities for academic departments of public health to engage in the reshaping of the agenda, particularly through working closely with primary care organizations and communities.

Conclusion

The rapid pace of change does not allow an assessment of whether the new structure will be more effective in improving the health of the population. The challenges for delivering improved public health include making health improvement a real priority for primary care, which may well be deflected to the acute services agenda, developing new and changing roles for a variety of staffs, and making a reality of the opportunities for working with government both at local and regional levels. There are anxieties about the adequacy of the public health capacity. Above all, national commitment is needed to invest in developing multidisciplinary public health professionals and to invest at all levels. Networks are embryonic and will be needed to maintain existing skills and create an accountability structure which delivers better population health. The major risks for public health specialists will come from the pace of change, potential fragmentation, stretched capacity, and lack of clear roles.

This chapter has described the current policy context within England, much of which is common across the United Kingdom. It has identified both the political policies and the specific plans which impact on the public's health and the way that the public health function is changing. The NHS, and national government policy in other areas, are committed to reducing health inequalities. The challenges to public health are to maintain its profile, to avoid becoming swamped either by the minutiae of organizational change or the dominance of the acute care agenda, and to utilize the opportunities, which undoubtedly exist.

References

[1] Department of Health. Independent Inquiry into Inequalities in Health, Chair: Sir Donald Acheson. London: HMSO, 1998.

[2] Goldblatt P, Davies S, Bissett B. *Are we living longer and in better health?* London: Office for National Statistics, 2001.

[3] Statistics Users Council, Annual Conference Report, London, Health and Care Statistics, 15 November 2001.

[4] Health Survey for England: *Methodology and documentation*, London: HMSO, 2000.

[5] Department of Health: *The Cancer Plan*. London: HMSO, 2000.

[6] Department of Health: *Saving Lives: Our Healthier Nation*, London: HMSO, 1999.

[7] Department of Health: *The NHS Plan*. London: HMSO, 2000.

[8] British Heart Foundation/New Opportunities Fund/National Countryside Agency: Walking the way to health scheme, London, 2000.

[9] Bartlett H, Ashley A, Howells K. *Evaluation of Sonning Common Health Walks Scheme*. Oxford: Oxford Brookes University, 1996.

[10] Banks P. *Partnerships under Pressure*. London: The Kings Fund, 2002.

[11] Social Exclusion Unit. *A new commitment to Neighbourhood Renewal: National Strategy and Action Plan*. London: HMSO, 2001.

[12] Social Exclusion Unit. *Sure Start Plus*. London, July 2000.

[13] Department of the Environment Transport and the Regions. *Second Report on the National Cycling Strategy*, London, 1999.

[14] The Home Office. *Crime and Disorder Act*. London, 1998.

[15] Lang T, Rayner G. *Why Health is the Key to the Future of Food and Farming*. London: Thames Valley University, 2002.

[16] House of Commons Select Committee, Second Report: public health 1 (session 2000-1): HC30-1.

[17] British Heart Foundation: Coronary heart disease statistics database 2002: Annual compendium: 2002 edition, BHF: London, 2002.

[18] Department of Health. *Tackling Health Inequalities: Consultation on a Plan for Delivery*. London: HMSO, 2001.

[19] Wanless D. Independent Review: *Securing our future health; taking a long term view*. HM Treasury, 2002.

[20] Secretary of State LSE Health Lecture by Alan Milburn. London, 8 March 2000.

[21] The Faculty of Public Health Medicine. *Ten key areas for specialist public health practice*. London, 2001.

[22] Department of Health. *Shifting the Balance of Power*. London: HMSO, 2001.

[23] Minister of Health. Lecture to public health specialists by Lord Phillip Hunt. London: The Kings Fund, 13 November 2001.

[24] Department of Health. *The Report of the CMO's project to Strengthen the Public Health Function*. London, 2001.

[25] Department of Health. *Getting Ahead of the Curve*. London: HMSO, 2002.

[26] The NHS Confederation. *Clinical Networks: a Discussion Paper*. London, 2001.

Chapter 4

Public health in Sweden: Facts, visions and lessons

Stig Wall, Gudrun Persson and
Lars Weinehall

Introduction

Sweden has a long tradition of public health reporting. Vital statistics and death cause registration were initiated in Sweden earlier than in any other European country by the Commission of Tables, founded in 1749. The Commission became the Central Bureau of Statistics in 1858 and is now Statistics Sweden [1]. From 1854 the provincial medical officers were required to submit annual reports on the health of their populations. Doctors were responsible for death certification in urban areas by 1860 and in rural areas by 1911 when a standardized cause of death list was established [2]. The broad population perspective on health issues, however, gradually fell into abeyance as a consequence of progress in medicine and continuing specialization.

A renewed public health interest from Swedish health authorities occurred during the 1970s with a changing perspective from medical care policy to health policy [3]. In 1984, in conjunction with the World Health Organization (WHO) "Health for All by the year 2000" strategy [4], a national Health Care Commission presented a model for systematic description of the population and its health risks, health problems and care facilities. As a consequence, the government proposed that a compilation and analysis of the health of the population should be published every third year. The task was undertaken by the National Board of Health and Welfare. Sweden's first national *Public Health Report* was published in 1987 [5].

This chapter examines the Swedish public health scene from three different perspectives, each of which involves different actors, public health *reporting*, public health *research*, and public health *policy*. By combining the three we emphasize their interdependence and provide some examples of successes and failures in Swedish health and welfare programmes.

Public health reporting is the responsibility of the Centre for Epidemiology within the National Board of Health and Welfare. The first report was published in 1987, the fifth in 2001 [6] and since 1994 Social Reports have been published in parallel [7]. These reports provide a basis for health and social policy and give a broad description and analysis of health and socioeconomic trends. They are used by national and local politicians and their organizations, health professionals, journalists, and by public health training programmes. Data from national registers, surveys of living conditions and work environments and labour force surveys provide the empirical basis for public health reporting. The Swedish personal identification number, a unique asset but also a matter of ethical concern, makes it possible to link health registers to census data, income registers and education registers. National legislation—The Personal Data Act—sets the rules for the ethical conduct and use of these data [8]. The Swedish Data Inspection Board—the supervisory authority—ensures that processing of personal data is in accordance with the law, securing personal integrity and public access to information.

Public health research in Sweden is often based on epidemiological population studies, for which the potential is especially great in Sweden because of the availability of central disease and population registers of good quality [9–11]. Considerable attention has been placed on the social "landscape" of diseases and their prevention. The first Public Health Report revealed that Sweden had substantial, and possibly widening, social gaps in health [5,12].

Public health policy in Sweden has not been subject to comprehensive national development. According to the Swedish constitution, health care has been mainly a regional responsibility. However, the perspective has widened and in 1997 the Swedish government appointed a National Committee to formulate national goals for public health and to suggest strategies for their achievement [13].

We now summarize the public health situation in Sweden as mirrored by its five national public health reports (1987–2001) and identify major themes in Swedish public health research and policy. We also describe the lessons learnt from trying to promote and evaluate public health change at the local community level.

Demographic and health trends

Life expectancy continues to increase

Life expectancy at birth increased by over twenty years for men and almost twenty-five years for women since 1900 to the present 77.5 years for men and 82.1 years for women. By international comparison, Sweden is well placed; only men in Iceland and Japan live longer. During the past few decades the length of men's lives has grown more quickly than that of women. The recent increases in life expectancy are due mainly to the decrease in mortality among middle-aged and older adults and particularly cardiovascular disease mortality, with men benefiting more than women. Together with the trend for women to give birth to fewer children, 1.5 children per woman in 2000—the lowest fecundity since the mid-nineteenth century, population growth is tapering off as the population ages (Fig. 4.1).

Infant mortality continues to decline

During the past fifteen years infant mortality has halved to a low of 3.4 deaths during the first year of life per 1000 live births. The decline in infant mortality during the past few decades has been more pronounced during the first month of life, while the opposite occurred during earlier periods. This shift is explained largely by improved neonatal care. During the 1970s and 1980s the number of cases of sudden infant death syndrome (SIDS) increased in Sweden as in many other countries. The situation later improved when increasing numbers of children were again sleeping on their backs, a successful nonmedical intervention [14]. During the 1990s the rate of SIDS deaths in Sweden declined rapidly and was down to 0.4 per 1000 live births in 1999.

Longer life—better health?

What then is the quality of the years added to life? According to an index developed by Statistics Sweden, it is chiefly years with slight ill health that have been added. A decrease in the number of "healthy" years has taken place mainly for the ages 16–44 years and particularly among women. Health development during the last two decades has favoured those aged forty-five or older rather than younger adults. Self-reported good health has improved most for men and women over sixty-five. This is paralleled by improved mobility and declining proportions of disabled and fewer with daily living difficulties, partly an effect of knee and hip arthroplasty. Vision has improved due to the large number of cataract operations. Dental health has also improved considerably. Mild mental problems such as anxiety and sleep problems are being reported less than formerly in this age group. For ages 16–44, the proportion that consider their health as good remained stable for most of the 1980s but gradually decreased during the 1990s. Mental ill health problems, such as anxiety, worry and sleep

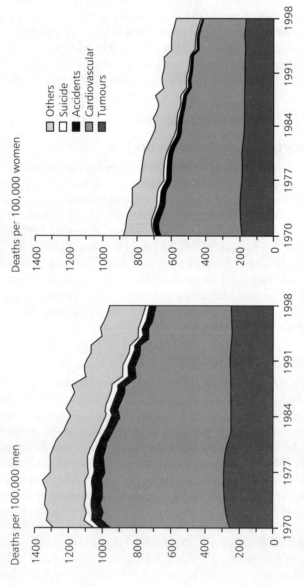

Fig. 4.1 Deaths per 100,000 from different causes 1978–1998. Age-standardized.
Source: Cause of Death Register, EpC/National Board of Health and Welfare.

problems, became more common during the 1990s in these age groups. This coincided with the economic depression during the first half of the 1990s when there was high unemployment in Sweden.

Cardiovascular disease—fewer new cases and more survivors

In less than two decades mortality from cardiovascular diseases in ages 15–74 has more than halved in Sweden due to reductions in incidence and case fatality; these declines have especially occurred among the well educated thus contributing to widening health inequalities [15]. However, during the 1990s, cardiovascular diseases still accounted for almost half of the total mortality.

The decreased risks of developing cardiovascular disease are due to improvements in the major risk factors, predominantly reduced smoking and improved dietary habits, while the reduced risks of dying are due largely to medical care efforts [6]. The proportion of daily smokers has been declining since about 1960 among men and since 1980 among women. In 1999, 18 percent of men and 19 percent of women aged 16–84 smoked daily compared with almost half of men in Estonia, and among women, a third in Denmark, Norway and the Netherlands and 7 percent in Russia and Portugal.

Inequalities in health

Produced or reproduced?

Several studies, often using a lifespan approach, have shown the importance of conditions early in life for health development [16]. Family conflicts, in particular, are predictive of later ill health and mortality, as is growing up in split families or in economic despair. These results refute the view that understanding of adult health is mainly to be found in adult living conditions. Socioeconomic conditions in childhood have also been shown to relate to attained height and the self-reported health as an adult, attained body height being a collective end result of social rather than nutritional conditions [17]. In northern Sweden, a longitudinal study of cardiovascular risk indicators confirms that the so-called metabolic syndrome (overweight, high serum cholesterol and insulin, elevated blood pressure) can be found among adolescents [18] and that the clustering of risk factors, especially smoking, is affected by social background, especially for girls [19]. Other studies, encouragingly, point to the benefits of physical activity among teenagers [20].

By combining information from national mortality registers, population registers and the so-called Level of Living Surveys, social stratification has been shown to operate from early life into old age and for perceived health, total and cause-specific mortality—cardiovascular in particular, and also for biological indicators such as height, gestational period and birth-weight [21,22]. Independently of these factors there are social differences in infant mortality and during childhood and adolescence there are also differences in mortality by parental social class, immigration and civil status. These patterns are general in respect of outcome and seem to forecast children's future health prospects. Thus, the social environment and the social career following school performance in childhood, predict self-reported health and cardiovascular disease in adulthood. Among older people, social differences exist in health, functional capacity, survival and mortality [23]. By means of the "conscript register," it has been possible to show how occupational choice and future ill health in young men are affected by social background, living conditions and physical capacity. Health-related selection to occupations and social classes operate [24] and risk factors are over-represented among men later belonging to the low socioeconomic classes and underrepresented among those men later belonging to the higher socioeconomic strata. Many risk factor patterns are established in adolescence and are strongly tied to educational level and future social class.

Widening gap?

A major obligation for public health practitioners is to increase the visibility of the social and gender differentials in health. The first Public Health Report [5] noted that:

> "although, during the 1970's material conditions equalized between people, class differences increased with regard to exposure for such living conditions that had health impacts, e.g., smoking, unemployment, stress and monotonous work."

Subsequent public health reports have found persistent social differences in health [6]. They are greatest among men; male upper white-collar workers at age thirty-five are expected to live two years longer than unskilled male blue-collar workers and female upper white-collar workers 0.7 years longer than female unskilled blue-collar workers.

A probable explanation of social differences in morbidity and mortality is that health risks cluster among individuals in certain social groups. Unhealthy living habits (including high energy intake that can lead to excess weight, smoking and high alcohol consumption) which are today more common among blue-collar workers, were previously more common among white-collar workers. One tenth of the population has an accumulation of welfare problems such as low income, economic problems, difficulties in obtaining employment, and problems on the housing market or low housing standards. They also report more health problems and unhealthy living habits which tend to accumulate among those who are socially exposed and vulnerable [6,7]. The same pattern of social differences is observed for different educational levels. The importance of education is further supported by the fact that educational advantage *within* all socioeconomic strata seems to be beneficial.

In relative mortality terms, the ratio of blue-collar workers to white-collar workers during the period 1990–1994 varies for European Union countries between 1.5 and 2.0 (Table 4.1). For Sweden it is up to 1.6, which is higher than in Denmark, Norway and England. Expressed in absolute numbers, blue-collar workers in Sweden have lower mortality than blue-collar workers in any other of the European countries studied [25]. Among white-collar workers too, Sweden had the lowest mortality measured as deaths per 100,000 persons and year. The generally lower death rate in Sweden means that even small absolute differences give higher relative differences in Sweden than in countries with higher death rates. The same absolute difference "weighs more heavily" at a lower level. From a social-equality perspective, it may be relevant to use absolute mortality or morbidity in the socially or economically worst-off groups as a comparative measure of how well countries are looking after their population's health [26].

Table 4.1 Deaths per 100,000 person-years by socioeconomic group in some European countries. Men 30–59 years. Periods 1990–1994

Country	Blue-collar	White-collar	Ratio
Sweden	410	250	1.6
Denmark	570	390	1.5
Finland	690	360	1.9
Norway	430	280	1.5
England and Wales	460	300	1.5
Ireland	540	320	1.7
Spain	510	260	2.0

Source: [25].

Public health policy in Sweden

A process

For the first time, Sweden is in the process of deciding on a comprehensive national public health policy which is expected to be adopted by the Parliament in 2002. The new policy aims to strengthen health promotion and disease prevention initiatives, contribute to a reduction of health inequalities between groups, and make health consequences an important consideration in all decision making at every level of society. The National Committee for Public Health was commissioned in 1997 to propose national goals for public health as well as strategies for achieving these goals. A number of experts and researchers within various areas collaborated on the development of these goals and nineteen different expert-produced reports were published (Fig. 4.2).

During the three years of its work the Committee fostered a broad discussion with the public and with politicians and civil servants at State and municipal level, with research workers, and with representatives of different organisations and trades. Furthermore, the Committee invited representatives of different organizations and popular movements to actively monitor the work.

Focusing on the determinants of health

As a basis for its proposals, the Commission used the series of national public health reports and when summarising the health trends, three

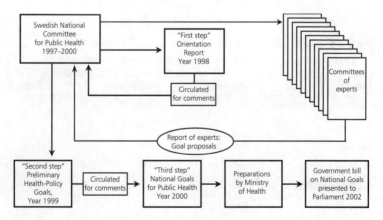

Fig. 4.2 The process of the National Public Health Committee—three steps towards the formulation of national goals

issues were important: the steadily increasing life expectancy; the pattern of declining self-estimated good health among young people; and the remaining health gap between different social strata. Contrary to many other national health policies, the Swedish health goals mainly address determinants of health [27]. The goals are directed to the level of society and culture and attempt to put health issues on the political as well as the social agenda [13]. The Swedish public health vision is aiming at good health for all on equal terms. Each individual should be allowed opportunities to achieve the best state of health possible: an environment is needed which promotes health for all while offering special support for those in need. The Committee has formulated six overall strategies, forming the basis for the national goals of public health:

* strengthening the social capital;
* growing-up in a satisfactory environment;
* improving conditions at work;
* creating a satisfactory physical environment;
* stimulating health-promoting life habits;
* developing a satisfactory infrastructure for health.

From these strategies eighteen public health goals were developed (Table 4.2). Some of the goals include initiatives to develop the social capital, to counteract wider disparities in income and reduce relative poverty, to give all children the opportunity to grow up on fair and safe terms, to support high employment, to create accessible areas for recreation and to promote safe environments and products. Other goals deal with preconditions for public health research and public health information, or aim at stronger collaborations at the local level, based on a new Public Health Law. The focus on life style factors (food, activities, drugs) should not "blame the individual", but support and facilitate healthier living. The importance of partnerships with health care providers is recognized and they are challenged to focus more on disease prevention and health promotion and to foster inter-sectoral work. The proposals aim to prevent ill health that restricts the freedom of the individual. Changes have to take place in the labour market, in welfare policy and in consumption patterns, as well as with regard to health care policy.

When assessing the goals, target groups should be defined and instructions for implementation should be issued to appropriate agencies. National public health policy should be co-ordinated by the Government. For national, regional and local authorities, as well as for private and voluntary sectors, a number of actions and challenges are defined. Monitoring

Table 4.2 The proposed eighteen goals for the Swedish National Public Health Policy

Goal 1
Strong solidarity and community cohesion
- Reduced poverty
- Reduced segregation in housing
- Support for socially disadvantaged children and adolescents

Goal 2
Supportive social environments
- Reduced isolation, loneliness and insecurity
- Increased participation in voluntary organisations and culture

Goal 3
Safe and equal growing-up conditions
- Safe and secure attachment between children and parents
- Promote health, self-confidence and achievements in schools
- Improved mental health among children and adolescents

Goal 4
High employment
- Good opportunities for life-long learning
- Low unemployment
- No labour market discrimination against immigrants and disabled

Goal 5
Good working environment
- Adaptation of demands to worker's individual capabilities
- Increased influence and opportunities for development
- Reduced overtime

Goal 6
Access to green open spaces for recreation
- Quiet and safe green open spaces easily accessible
- Stimulating school yard-environments

- Good outdoor environment for home nursing and the disabled

Goal 7
Healthy indoor and outdoor environments
- Reduced exposure to environmental tobacco smoke
- Well ventilated indoor environment
- Well-planned housing environment, safe radiation environment, fresh air and non-toxic environment

Goal 8
Safe environments and products
- Safe housing and traffic and public environments
- Reduced use of health hazardous and allergy inducing products

Goal 9
Increased physical activity
- Increased physical activities in schools and at work
- Increased physical activities during recreational time

Goal 10
Healthy food habits
- Increased consumption of fruits and vegetables and decreased consumption of fats and sugar
- Reduced prevalence of overweight in the population
- Increased prevalence of breast-feeding

Goal 11
Safe and secure sexuality
- Decreased transmission of sexually transmitted infections
- Reduced prevalence of undesired pregnancies
- No discrimination against people due to their sexual preferences

Table 4.2 *continued*

Goal 12
Decreased tobacco use
– A tobacco-free start in life from the
  year 2010
– By the year 2010, a 50 percent
  reduction of adolescents under
  18 who start smoking or using
  wet snuff
– By the year 2010, a 50 percent
  reduction of smokers among
  groups that smoke the most
– Nobody shall unwillingly be exposed
  to smoke in their
  environment

Goal 13
Reduction of harmful use of alcohol
– Reduced total consumption
– Complete abstinence during
  pregnancy, at the workplace, at
  sports and fitness activities, and in
  connection with road and sea traffic
– Reduced binge drinking

Goal 14
A drug-free society
– Reduced supply of narcotics
– Reduced number of adolescents
  trying and using drugs

Goal 15
A more health-promoting health
service
– Foster interventions at individual,
  group and population levels
– Increased collaboration to foster
  equal health development

– Developed methods and strategies
  for disease prevention and
  health promotion

Goal 16
Co-ordinated public health work
– Responsibility for health planning at
  a municipal and county
  council level
– Development of co-ordinated
  multi-sectorial public health
  strategies at a national level by
  concerned national public agencies
– Co-ordination of public health
  policies in the Swedish Cabinet
  Office and the Ministries
– Periodical National Public Health
  Policy report to the Parliament

Goal 17
Long-term investment in research,
development of methods and
education
– Intensified research on the
    usefulness, costs and
    consequences
  of intervention methods in public
  health
– Improved methods for public health
  work
– Increased educational investment in
  public health sciences

Goal 18
Objective health information
– Access to objective and impartial
  health information

and evaluation of the national public health goals are to be reported to the Government every five years in two reports: one on public health policy from the National Institute of Public Health and the other as part of the National Public Health Report from the National Board of Health and Welfare.

Lessons from a public health intervention program: The Norsjö case

Epidemiological studies from the late 1970s showed that the county of Västerbotten had the highest cardiovascular mortality in Sweden [3] and as a result a long-term prevention program, the Västerbotten Intervention Program, was initiated in 1985. The community intervention in Norsjö— the municipality with the highest mortality—combined individual and population-oriented efforts. Popular movement activities in the community brought ideas out into the public. Contrary to other models, the health sector and its primary health care providers took an active role in the work [28,29]. All individuals at ages thirty, forty, fifty, and sixty were invited to participate in an educational screening including health counselling (Fig. 4.3). In the 10-year evaluation the intervention area had a significantly larger decline in cholesterol, systolic blood pressure and predicted coronary disease (CHD) mortality [30]. Lower educated people seemed to benefit the most from the prevention program (Fig. 4.3).

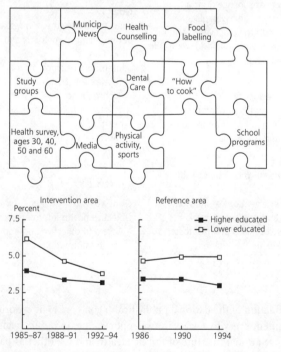

Fig. 4.3 Components in the Norsjö intervention and the estimated risk of dying of cardiac infarction in comparison with northern Sweden (reference area) stratified by educational level

Future scenarios

A governmental task force recently presented its *"Balance Sheet for Welfare of the 1990s"* in terms of health, education, work, economy, social security and relations, and political resources [31]. Major negative changes are seen for the decade, as have been documented in the previous public health and social reports. These changes are occurring while death rates have continued to drop, infant mortality has halved and education levels improved even further. Especially vulnerable groups are lone mothers with meagre economical resources, immigrants with declining social positions, and young people increasingly experiencing perceived ill health and social insecurity.

People in Sweden will continue to be healthier than earlier generations and the future disease patterns will be dominated by the problems associated with ageing. Mortality rates will continue to decrease for many causes. Paradoxically, however, reduced risks along with medical care successes are creating new medical care problems. If tobacco and alcohol consumption decline, and eating and activity patterns continue to improve, then the disease risks will be reduced. However, despite general improvements in both food and exercise habits, the proportion of overweight people has increased. Expected lower alcohol prices in the future will lead to increased alcohol consumption and more alcohol-related injuries. In general, there is no indication that serious mental disease is on the increase, rather the reverse; however, many people experience increased worry and anxiety, partly because of increased stress in working life [6]. The number of persons living with cancer has increased greatly in Sweden [32]. The decline in cardiovascular diseases may continue if current risk factor trends prevail, or the disease trends may be counteracted by the increasing overweight problem.

Children and young people in Sweden have long had a very favorable health development although there are several disturbing trends, for example the increase in juvenile diabetes [33]. The effects of unemployment in younger ages for later somatic and mental health problems, as well as alcohol and tobacco consumption, have been documented [34].

Lessons for public health

Swedish research supports the view that work and other living conditions interact with other early risk factors to produce and reproduce health inequalities. How then do we respond to the challenge of the social differences? Since social inequality is manifested through the accumulation of risk factors during life among vulnerable groups, prevention should focus on the social situation rather than on the individual risk factors. We still lack basic knowledge on how people in different social positions take advantage of and adopt society's well-meant health messages, for example, on lifestyle changes. A Swedish Enquiry into Democracy and Power [35] emphasized that the well educated are sure to take advantage of the opportunities. They take the lead as early adopters [36] and eventually others follow. Should the widening social gap be interpreted as a result of the general and unspecific structure of public heath policy? Does equity in health in fact call for an unequal prevention approach? And what lessons for health policy could be learnt from the well documented inequalities in health between and within countries and from the observations that an unequal society in itself is a risk factor over and above that of the individual's social position?

The point of departure for several studies comparing Sweden with other countries has been the hypothesis that our social policy and relative social homogeneity should yield less of health inequity. The underlying mechanism behind social inequality in health, however, is probably more related to fundamental issues than to short-term health and social policy. More decisive changes require a sustainable policy [37]. Others suggest that equality has become politically outdated [38] and identify the ethical principle of autonomy as a hindrance for policy in that it prevents the targeting of vulnerable groups [39]. Public health work should not add to risks and needs to establish its ethical platform. We need an evidence-based public health policy; this implies that we must also be prepared to analyze the health consequences of the many structural interventions imposed by current welfare politics [40].

It is time to act in accordance with what we know about the social circumstances beyond individual control—the evidence on social inequalities is overwhelming and needs no further documentation [41]. What is needed is a committed policy and local interventions for social and behavioral change involving the community. Evaluations of such actions must focus on structure and process as well as outcome and discuss measures and criteria of success not only in disease terms but also areas such as cultural and democratic development, and psychological and emotional well being. We need to move beyond analysing the impact of social factors on health to documenting the contribution of health and health care to society and economic development [42].

Although public health research in Sweden is widely known to be multi-disciplinary, it is mainly hosted by the medical faculties and its scope has been widened to include the functioning and quality of the health care as well as its role as a partner in preventive work. The research agenda on social inequalities in health has, to a large extent, been set by medical sociologists and epidemiologists. The recognized importance of the field is shown by a governmental commission to develop a national research program to counteract social inequalities in health [12] and by the recent establishment of a center and network for research on health equity. This research is now moving from describing these gaps to attempts at understanding the mechanisms behind the stratification. In congruence with the increasing demands for health interventions, there is a parallel need for research on the benefits from such interventions. There is a considerable gap between the epidemiological identification of risk factors and the documentation of the effects of intervention. There is an epidemiological potential in prevention and a challenge lies in bringing the development of epidemiological theory nearer to public health efforts. This calls for conceptual and methodological development of evaluations of public health interventions, not only of their efficacy but also in terms of cost-effectiveness, social acceptance and ethical consequences. Medical practice also needs a clearer public health perspective in everyday work [13].

To make objective health information accessible to all [13], it is important to research the area of communication between those who generate public health knowledge and those who will use it [43]. When complicated situations and uncertain causal mechanisms are simplified at the same time as conflicting scientific conclusions are broadcast in the mass media, confidence in public health will be affected.

The potential, limitations and frustrations of collaborative research have been described [44]. Global health problems are rarely covered in traditional public health textbooks, despite the fact that methodological issues are even more important in situations where health problems are great and resources are scarce. Global public health knowledge is fostered by work across disciplines and cultures. International collaboration in research and training can be a lever for mutual understanding and eventually for beneficial social and economic change.

References

[1] Documents of Death Cause Statistics. *Hygiea* 1856; **18**: 798–817.

[2] Luther G. The Birth of Official Statistics in 18th Century Sweden. In: *Bull International Statistical Institute*, 52nd Session, Finland, 1999; available at www.stat.fi/isi99.

[3] Rosén M. *Epidemiology in Planning for Health—with special reference to regional epidemiology and the use of health registers.* Umeå university Medical Dissertations New Series No 188. ISSN 0346-6612. Umeå1987.

[4] Global Strategy for Health by the year 2000. Geneva: World Health Organization, 1981.

[5] Public Health Report 1987. The National Board of Health and Welfare. Stockholm, 1987.

[6] Persson G, Boström G, Diderichsen F et al. (eds.). Health in Sweden— The National Public Health Report 2001. *Scand J Public Health* 2001; **29** (Suppl 58).

[7] Social Report 2001. The National Board of Health and Welfare. Stockholm, 2001.

[8] Allebeck P. The Helsinki declaration: Good for patients? Good for public health? *Scand J Public Health* 2002; **30**: 1–4.

[9] Wall S, Källestål C. *Epidemiology Research in Sweden—Structure, Conditions and Need—A Task Force Report*. Swedish Medical and Social Research Councils. ISBN 91-88758-16-18, 1996.

[10] Evaluation of Swedish Epidemiological Research. Swedish Council for Social Research. ISBN 91-88758-23-0, 1997.

[11] Rosén M. National health Data Registers—A Nordic heritage to public health. *Scand J Public Health* 2002; **30**: 81–5.

[12] Promoting Research on Inequality in Health. Swedish Council for Social Research ISBN 91-88758-28-1, 1998.

[13] Health on Equal Terms—national goals for public health. Final report by the Swedish National Committee for Public Health. *Scand J Public Health* 2001; **29** (Suppl 57).

[14] Högberg U, Bergström E. Suffocated Prone: The iatrogenic tragedy of SIDS. *Am J Public Health* 2000; **90**: 527–31.

[15] Tunstall-Pedoe H, Kuulasmaa K, Mahonen M et al. Contribution of trends in survival and coronary-event rates to changes in coronary heart disease mortality: 10-year results from 37 WHO MONICA project populations. Monitoring trends and determinants in cardiovascular disease. *Lancet* 1999; **353**: 1547–57.

[16] Lundberg O. The impact of childhood living conditions on illness and mortality in adulthood. *Soc Sci Med* 1993; **36**: 1047–52.

[17] Nyström Peck M, Lundberg O. Short stature as an effect of economic and social conditions in childhood. *Soc Sci Med* 1995; **41**: 733–8.

[18] Bergström E, Hernell O, Persson LÅ, Vessby B. Insulin resistance syndrome in adolescents. *Metabolism* 1996; **45**: 908–14.

[19] Bergström E, Hernell O, Persson LÅ. Cardiovascular risk indicators cluster in girls from families of low socio-economic status. *Acta Paediatr* 1996; **85**: 1083–90.

[20] Barnekow-Bergkvist M. Physical capacity, physical activity and health—a population based fitness study of adolescents with an 18-year follow-up. Umeå university Medical Dissertations New Series No 494, 1997.

[21] Nyström-Peck M. Childhood class, body weight and adult health. Doctoral thesis. Stockholm: Institute for Social Research, 1994.

[22] Östberg V. The social patterning of child mortality: the importance of social class, gender, family structure, immigrant status and population density. *Sociol Health Illness* 1997; **19**: 415–35.

[23] Vågerö D, Lundberg O. Socio-economic differentials among adults in Sweden—towards an explanation. In: Lopez A, Valkmen T, Caselli G. (eds.). *Premature Adult Mortality in Developed Countries*. Oxford: Oxford University Press, 1995.

[24] Hemmingsson T, Lundberg I, Nilsson R, Allebeck P. Health related selection to seafaring occupations and its effects on morbidity and mortality. *Am J Ind Med* 1997; **31**: 662–8.

[25] Kunst AE, Groenhof F, Andersen O et al. Occupational class and ischemic heart disease mortality in the United States and 11 European countries. *Am J Public Health* 1999; **89**: 47–53.

[26] Vågerö D, Eriksson R. Socioeconomic inequalities in morbidity and mortality in western Europe. Correspondence. *Lancet* 1997; **350**: 516–17.

[27] Pearson TA. Scandinavia's lessons to the world of public health. *Scand J Public Health* 2000; **28**: 161–3.

[28] Weinehall L, Westman G, Hellsten G et al. Shifting the distribution of risk: Results of a community intervention in a Swedish programme for the prevention of Cardiovascular disease. *J Epidemiol and Comm Health* 1999; **53**: 243–50.

[29] Weinehall L. Partnership for health. On the role of primary health care in a community intervention programme. Umeå University Medical Dissertations, New Series No 531, Umeå Sweden, 1997.

[30] Weinehall L, Hellsten G, Boman K et al. Can a sustainable community intervention reduce the health gap? 10-year evaluation of a Swedish community intervention program for the prevention of cardiovascular disease. *Scand J Public Health* 2001; **29** (Suppl 56): 59–68.

[31] Välfärdsbokslut för 1990-talet (*Balance Sheet for Welfare of the 1990's*) Statens Offentliga Utredningar SOU 2001:79. Stockholm 2001.

[32] Stenbeck M, Rosén M, Sparén P. Causes of increasing cancer prevalence in Sweden. *Lancet* 1999; **354**: 1093–4.

[33] Dahlquist G, Mustonen L. Analysis of 20 years of prospective registration of childhood onset diabetes—time trends and birth cohort effects. *Acta Paediatr* 2000; **89**: 1231–7.

[34] Hammarström A, Janlert U. Nervous and depressive symptoms in a longitudinal study of youth unemployment—selection or exposure? *J Adolesc* 1997; **20**: 293–305.

[35] *Demokrati och Makt i Sverige*. Maktutredningens huvudrapport (*Democracy and Power in Sweden*: The Main Report of the Power Enquiry). Stockholm: SOU;1990:44. (In Swedish).

[36] Pearson TA, Wall S, Lewis C et al. Dissecting the "black box" of community intervention: Lessons from community-wide cardiovascular disease

prevention programs in the US and Sweden. *Scand J Public Health* 2001; **29** (Suppl 56): 69–78.

[37] Vågerö D. Health inequalities—searching for causal explanations. In: *Inequality in Health—A Swedish Perspective*. Stockholm: Swedish Council for Social Research, 1998.

[38] Lindbladh E, Lyttkens CH, Hanson BS, Östergren PO. Equity is out of fashion? An essay on autonomy and health policy in the individualized society. *Soc Sci Med* 1998; **46**: 1017–25.

[39] Lindbladh E, Lyttkens CH, Hanson BS et al. An economic and sociological interpretation of social differences in health-related behaviour: an encounter to guide social epidemiology. *Soc Sci Med* 1996; **43**: 1817–25.

[40] Wall S. Epidemiology in transition. *Int J Epidemiol* 1999; **28**: S1000–S1004.

[41] Krasnik A, Rasmussen NK (eds.). Reducing social inequalities in health—evidence, policy and practice. *Scand J Public Health* 2002; **30** (Suppl 59): 1–5.

[42] Yach D. Economics and public health. Reflections from the past, challenges for the future. *Scand J Public Health* 2001; **29**: 241–4.

[43] Wall S. Epidemiology for prevention. *Int J Epidemiol* 1995; **24**: 655–64.

[44] Wall S. Public health research cooperation and capacity building—some experiences from a longterm North-South venture. *Eur J Public Health* 2000; **10**: 7–10.

Chapter 5

Public health in eastern Europe and the former Soviet Union

Martin McKee and Witold Zatonski

Patterns of health; the same but different

In the post-war period, while many aspects of life in western Europe changed beyond recognition progress in eastern Europe was much slower. Between 1945 and 1990 the countries in the communist bloc shared an experience that continues to have profound implications for the health of their populations, as well as their ability to respond to them, more than ten years after the Soviet Union ceased to exist. The Soviet regime was isolated from the west by physical barriers, most obviously the Berlin Wall, but there was an equally important cultural divide. Yet this region is also very diverse, politically, geographically, and culturally [1].

Nonetheless, some simplification is possible. Politically, the region divides into two parts; those countries that were part of the Soviet Union and those that were its satellites (although for completeness this chapter will also consider two countries whose fate was intimately linked to the Soviet bloc, while not actually part of it, Yugoslavia and Albania). These political divisions are mirrored, to a surprising extent, in patterns of health (Fig. 5.1). Taking life expectancy at birth, with all its limitations as a broad summary measure, both parts of the Soviet bloc had attained a level broadly similar to the average for western Europe by the mid-1960s. Soon after, however, things began to go wrong. While life expectancy in western Europe steadily increased, in the countries of central and eastern Europe (CCEE) outside the Soviet Union it stagnated so that, by 1990, it was six years behind that in the west. In the Soviet Union, in contrast, life expectancy actually deteriorated, falling by two years between 1970 and

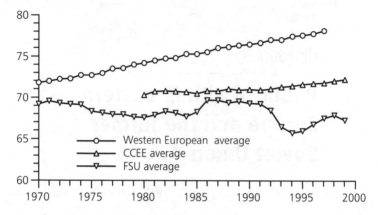

Fig. 5.1 Life expectancy at birth, in years (Source: WHO Health for All database)

1980. It then began a series of unexpected fluctuations in which life expectancy improved dramatically in 1985 before falling back after 1987 and then accelerating downwards. This pattern was relatively consistent across the fifteen republics that made up the Soviet Union, the exceptions being the more traditional central Asian Republics and Georgia.

In the period since 1990, the more "western" of the CCEE, such as Poland [2], the Czech Republic [3], and the former German Democratic Republic [4], have experienced rapid improvements in life expectancy while the more "eastern" ones, such as Romania and Bulgaria, are only now beginning to see some improvement. In the countries of the former Soviet Union (FSU) the path followed by each country was initially much more consistent, with a rapid fall in life expectancy until 1994, followed by a recovery which, in some such as Russia and Ukraine, peaked in 1998. One of the few exceptions to this pattern was Belarus, which after 1994 continued on a downward path. Belarus also differs from its neighbors in retaining a model of government that is little changed from the Soviet period and so, in broad terms, might be considered as acting as a control, showing what may have happened in its neighbors had the Soviet Union not ceased to exist.

Despite its many drawbacks, the Soviet regime bequeathed to epidemiologists a high quality system of vital statistics [5]. Some countries did conceal data at various times, either withholding data completely, as the Soviet Union did in the early 1980s, or "losing" certain sensitive causes such as homicide, suicide and cirrhosis in nonspecific categories, as occurred in the German Democratic Republic in the 1970s and 1980s. However, in all cases comprehensive mortality data sets have now been reconstructed [6]. The few remaining problems relate to coverage in some of the least developed parts of central Asia [7] and to regions afflicted by war, in the Caucasus [8] and the Balkans [9], where systems of vital regis-tration systems have been weakened but, more importantly, where the scale of migration is largely unrecorded.

A conceptual framework

To try to make sense of the patterns of health in this region, this chapter will take a systems approach [10]. Nearly all of the Soviet republics experi-enced a dramatic increase in life expectancy in 1985 and, perhaps more surprisingly as they were by then all independent, a steep fall between 1991 and 1994. Several distinct, and apparently unrelated causes of death con-tributed to these changes, such as injuries and heart disease, but not can-cer, indicating a phenomenon that must have its origins at a societal level, acting through multiple biological and social pathways. To add to the complexity, another perspective is necessary, that of time [11]. An under-standing of patterns of health in a population must also take account of the growing body of evidence linking circumstances in utero or in early childhood to health in later life, so that deaths today, for example from stroke or stomach cancer, reflect conditions several decades ago [12].

A first step—describing patterns of mortality

In this section the pragmatic separation of the CCEE and FSU will be maintained, reflecting their quite different experience of mortality although, as will be seen later, there are also certain common factors, in particular in relation to mechanisms of disease. Mortality can be disaggreg-ated in many ways. Looking first at gender, it is apparent that men have been especially vulnerable [13]. In all industrialized countries men have a lower life expectancy than women but the gap is especially large in the CCEE and FSU (Fig. 5.2).

Deaths among infants and young children have fallen steadily through-out the 1970s and 1980s, a decline that accelerated in the 1990s. There are a few exceptions, for example Romania, as a consequence of the policy adopted in the late 1980s of giving blood transfusions to many undernour-ished children who had been abandoned in "orphanages".[14] Death rates among older people are now generally higher than they were in 1990 in the FSU, although the difference is small in the three Baltic Republics. They are also slightly higher in the "eastern" CCEE, Romania, and Bulgaria, but have fallen in the "western" countries, such as Poland and the Czech Republic.

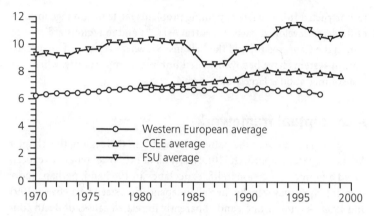

Fig. 5.2 Female–male difference in life expectancy (years) (Source: WHO Health for All database)

However the greatest impact has been on deaths in early middle age. Among the CCEE, deaths in this age group increased steadily throughout the 1980s. Subsequently, each country has experienced an improvement, but beginning at different times. In Poland and the Czech Republic it began almost at once while in Hungary and Bulgaria it only started in the mid-1990s. In Romania it was delayed until 1997. This age group was also affected most in the FSU, with their deaths driving the large fluctuations in overall mortality [15].

These changes have led to overall death rates among middle-aged men being about four times higher in the FSU than in western Europe; the difference between the CCEE and western Europe is about 2.5 times. Among women the differences are somewhat smaller and do not exhibit the peak at middle age seen among men. Death rates at older ages among both men and women in the CCEE and FSU are about twice those in western Europe.

The causes of death underlying these changes are extremely complex and the following description is, of necessity, a simplification. In the CCEE, most countries experienced a short-lived increase in deaths at the time of transition, largely due to deaths from external causes, especially traffic accidents, which have subsequently declined steadily during the remaining years of the 1990s [16]. Later, sustained improvements in life expectancy, beginning at different times in the 1990s, have largely been due to falls in cardiovascular disease. In some cases such as Poland, life expectancy has risen quite steeply [2]; in some parts of southern Europe, where rates were previously extremely high, a decline in deaths from cirrhosis has also contributed.

To understand the very different trends in the Soviet Union it is necessary to go back to events in 1985, when the Secretary General of the Communist party of the Soviet Union, Mikhail Gorbachev, implemented an initially highly effective and wide ranging anti-alcohol campaign [17]. This led to an immediate improvement in life expectancy, due largely to a decline in cardiovascular diseases and injuries. Smaller contributions were made by a range of causes known to be associated with alcohol, including acute alcohol poisoning and pneumonia. Importantly, other major causes of death, such as cancer, were unaffected. In the subsequent large fluctuations in mortality the same causes have been implicated, pointing to a major role for alcohol in the changing pattern of mortality in the former Soviet Union [18]. This issue is discussed in more detail below.

The immediate causes

A few specific conditions emerge as major causes of the health gap with western Europe: injuries and violence, cardiovascular disease, cancer, and some alcohol-related diseases such as cirrhosis.

Injuries and violence (external causes)

By 1997 the death rate from external causes was about four times higher in the FSU than in the west; in central and eastern Europe it was almost double that in the west. While all causes of injury are more common in this region than in the west, the gap is particularly great for homicide and suicide. Other external causes of death that are very much more common in the east than the west are drowning and deaths in fires.

Alcohol emerges as one common factor. In Russia, where these deaths have received most attention, deaths from all groups of external causes, and specific other causes, correlate closely with deaths from alcohol poisoning [19–21]. It is important to understand why people drink to excess. In Russia the highest rates of deaths from external causes, of all types, have been in those areas experiencing the most rapid pace of social and economic change [19]. This factor is common to deaths from many causes and it will be considered in more detail later in this chapter.

Death rates from unintentional injuries reflect many factors related to risk and its perception, and to the environment. Especially in the FSU, there are few of the design features that enhance safety in the west. In many cases effective health care could save some of these lives but it is either unavailable or of poor quality, especially in rural areas suffering from poor communications and transport infrastructure.

Cardiovascular disease

Deaths from cardiovascular disease are also much more common in eastern Europe than in the west. In central and eastern Europe this clearly reflects high levels of many traditional risk factors, such as a diet rich in saturated fats and high rates of smoking. In Poland there has been a marked decline in deaths from cardiovascular disease since the transition that is believed to reflect a change in the composition of fat in the diet [22] following removal of subsidies and the opening of the retail sector to international trade.

Trends in cardiovascular disease in the FSU have, however, presented epidemiologists with more of a puzzle. In the FSU, on several occasions death rates have changed substantially from one year to the next and death rates are especially high among the young. Deaths are also more likely to be sudden [23], with many victims showing little evidence of coronary atheroma at post mortem [24]. The conventional risk factors, such as lipid levels, and physical activity, identified in western epidemiological research, have little predictive value [25]. There is also evidence of differences in biochemical mechanisms [26].

The emphasis, in western epidemiology, on the role of lipids has distracted attention from the other elements of thrombosis, first described by Virchow over a century ago [27]. These include changes in vascular endothelium, permitting lipid to accumulate, and changes in platelet and fibrinolytic activity, influencing the propensity of blood to clot [28]. Eastern European diets characterized by large quantities of fat and very low levels of fruit and vegetables [29]. Correspondingly, antioxidant activity in blood, which is determined primarily by intake of micronutrients, is extremely low [30]. While changes in lipids are important, these other mechanisms may provide an explanation for rapidity of the reduction in cardiovascular deaths seen in some countries such as Poland [2] and the Czech Republic [3].

However these mechanisms cannot explain all of the observed effects, and in particular the much higher rate of sudden cardiac death among young men. Here it is likely that alcohol is playing an important role. In all of northern Europe, but especially in Russia and its neighbors, alcohol is typically drunk as vodka and in binges [31], unlike the more steady consumption in southern and western Europe. Reanalysis of studies looking at the cardiovascular effects of alcohol consumption found clear evidence that episodic heavy drinking, identified in various ways including frequent hangovers or getting into trouble with the police or frequent absence from work for alcohol related disorders, was consistently associated with a substantially increased risk of, especially, sudden cardiac death [32]. Other work has disentangled the physiological basis for these findings, showing very different responses of lipids, blood clotting and myocardial function to binge drinking and regular moderate consumption [33].

On the basis of what is known about the aetiology of cardiovascular disease in the west it is, however, unlikely that these explanations will be able to account for all of the changes that have been observed. Work from the Whitehall study, in particular, has highlighted the importance of psychosocial factors and there is also some evidence from this region to link stress and lack of control over events with cardiovascular disease [34].

Cancer

Cancer covers a multitude of diseases each with their own risk factors; here we consider two examples, lung and cervical cancer. Smoking has been extremely common among men in all of eastern Europe [35,36], possibly encouraged by a shared experience of military service as teenagers. Consequently, death rates from lung cancer among men are extremely high, in some cases reaching levels never previously observed anywhere in the world [37]. Interestingly, death rates from lung cancer are presently falling in many former Soviet countries but cohort analysis shows that this will be short lived, reflecting transiently lower levels of commencing smoking in the austere period of the late 1940s and early 1950s [38].

In contrast, smoking has always been relatively uncommon among women. This is now changing, and female smoking rates, especially among young women in major cities, are increasing rapidly, encouraged by aggressive advertising by western tobacco companies [39]. Consequently, lung cancer rates among women can soon be expected to start rising [40].

The policy response to tobacco has been, in general, very weak. The tobacco industry has been able to ignore health ministries with limited capacity that is stretched further by a focus on health care reform. Even where advertising is illegal, fines are often derisory. There are some exceptions. Poland has been able to implement a wide-ranging policy on tobacco [41], including a ban on advertising, that has led to a reduction in tobacco use. Such examples are, however, rare.

Cervical cancer is also somewhat more common than in the west, a finding that is unsurprising given the high rates of sexually transmitted diseases and, until recently, the difficulty in obtaining barrier contraceptives [42]. Unfortunately, the few effective cervical screening programmes are rare exceptions and screening is often opportunistic, with little quality control, and generally ineffective.

In brief, the pattern of cancer mortality in eastern Europe is complex and changing. In the future, it is likely that deaths from some types, such as stomach cancer, will continue to decline while others, such as breast and prostate, will come closer to those in the west.

Infectious diseases

As in the west, acute infectious disease is no longer one of the leading causes of death. This reflected the high level political commitment to disease control during the twentieth century, following Lenin's famous statement in response to outbreaks of typhus that "If communism does not destroy the louse, the louse will destroy communism". The Soviet system was especially successful in reducing vaccine preventable diseases, in part because of its pervasive system of monitoring and use of compulsion, although a breakdown of control systems in some countries following independence has allowed them to re-emerge [43]. In contrast, the lack of investment in infrastructure, with many rural hospitals lacking hot water even in the early 1990s, meant that other aspects of infection control were poor. This was exacerbated by adherence to outdated concepts of disease transmission and surveillance.

The other infectious diseases causing concern are sexually transmitted diseases (STDs), HIV, and tuberculosis. Rates of STDs rose rapidly in many countries in the 1990s. They have since fallen although there are concerns as to whether this reflects a true reduction in incidence or a decline in notification, as treatment is increasingly provided privately [44]. Rates of HIV infection are still low, in global terms, but are rising extremely quickly in many parts of the former Soviet Union [45]. At present, spread is primarily due to needle sharing among addicts but the epidemic is beginning to move into the wider population by means of sexual spread.

Rates of tuberculosis have also increased markedly in the 1990s with death rates returning to levels last seen in 1980. Rates are especially high among the large prison population, where conditions are highly conducive to rapid spread and where treatment is often inadequate [46]. A matter of particular concern is the high rate of drug resistant disease [47]. The co-existence of HIV and resistant tuberculosis poses enormous challenges for the future, and which have yet to elicit an effective response.

Finally, changes in land use, related to the adoption of new agricultural practices and a relaxation of earlier restraints on planning is contributing to a shift in patterns of zoonotic infections, such as an increase in leptospirosis in Bulgaria [48] and in tick-borne encephalitis in the Baltic states [49].

The underlying factors

One of the most striking features of mortality in eastern Europe is the way that men have been affected much more than women. This chapter argues that much of this can be explained in differences in lifestyle, in particular use of alcohol and tobacco. This is consistent with research on those rare populations where the gender gap in mortality is small [50,51].

Lifestyle choices are heavily influenced by social circumstances and they can only be understood fully by considering the context in which they are made. The social forces driving trends in mortality in this region are still inadequately understood, although some parts of the picture are clear. Those groups that have been worst affected have been so as a result of increasing deaths from external causes and cardiovascular diseases. Consistent with the findings discussed earlier, while deaths from causes linked directly with alcohol have been numerically less important, they have shown the steepest social gradients [52].

The rise in mortality has been the greatest in regions experiencing the most rapid pace of transition, as measured by gains and losses in employment [19], and where measures of social cohesion were weakest [53]. The individuals most affected have been men, with low levels of education [54], low levels of social support (such as the unmarried [55]) and low levels of control over their lives [56]. Women, Watson has argued [57], may have had some degree of protection as they could find fulfilling roles within the home while men with low skills levels were confronted with a feeling of impotence in a hostile and unresponsive world [58].

These findings paint a picture of societies in which young and middle-aged men in particular face a world of social and economic disruption that they are poorly prepared for [59]. For many, the opportunities are constrained by low levels of education and a lack of social support. Poor nutrition and high rates of smoking have already reduced their chances of a long life but the easy availability of cheap alcohol provides a pathway to oblivion and then to premature death. The hazards of drunkenness are exacerbated in a society in which there are few on whom one can depend and where one is surrounded by a poorly maintained, hazard-ridden environment.

The contribution of health care

There is now considerable evidence that timely and effective health care interventions have played an important role in reductions in mortality in western countries [60]. Research using the concept of avoidable mortality, has suggested that about 25 percent of the mortality gap between east and west Europe between birth and age seventy-five could be attributed to inadequacies in medical care in 1988 [61], with deaths from avoidable causes declining at a slower rate in the east than in the west.

While evidence of the contribution of health care to population health remains fragmentary, three broad patterns can be discerned within this region. Some countries, most often those that have been most successful in achieving economic growth, have been able to reform their health care systems relatively successfully. In others, mostly in the less developed parts of the FSU, while the basic infrastructure remains in place, some elements have effectively collapsed. In particular, there have been major problems with pharmaceutical supply. The third pattern is seen in those regions that have suffered from war and other conflict, where there has been widespread destruction of facilities and where what health care exists is often dependent on international development assistance [62].

While the specific impact of health care on measures of population health is often difficult to detect, there are several well-documented examples of where this has been identified [63,64]. Research on neonatal mortality has sought to separate the impact of health care from broader social determinants, with the former assessed by birth-weight specific survival and the latter by the overall birth weight distribution. In both the Czech Republic [65] and the former German Democratic Republic [66] there have been considerable improvements in birth-weight specific mortality, and by implication, the quality of care. As a consequence, closing the remaining gap with the best performing western countries will require policies that address the social determinants of low birth-weight.

In the second group of countries the situation is much less satisfactory. It is likely that the increase in mortality among the elderly in some FSU countries is a consequence of a reduction in the quality of health care, especially as the increase is greatest, and more sustained, in countries such as Belarus where the economic situation is worst. However the main evidence is from deaths among young people with diabetes. This population is especially susceptible to a breakdown in the delivery of health care; in the absence of a regular supply of insulin, they will simply die. Deaths from diabetes at ages under fifty increased about eightfold in the 1990s in many former Soviet countries [67].

The collapse in vital registration systems that has accompanied the breakdown of health care delivery in areas beset by conflict means that there is very little information available. It is almost certain that, apart from the more obvious direct effects of war, there will have been a substantial increase in mortality among those with chronic diseases requiring long term treatment, including not only diabetes and hypertension but also conditions such as asthma and epilepsy.

The public health response

The public health challenges facing policy makers in this region are enormous. So why has the public health response been so weak? An earlier analysis of the policy inaction on childhood injuries provides some clues [68]. One problem was that worsening health was invisible. Data on health trends presented to politicians is often limited to easily understood aggregate measures, such as life expectancy at birth. While this has the benefit of simplicity it obscures the complex nature of mortality. In the CCEE in the 1980s it was recognized that life expectancy was stagnating but this concealed a substantial increase in mortality among young and middle-aged men, which was counteracted by a steady fall in infant mortality [69].

A second problem was a lack of public health capacity. Organizations responsible for public health were typically weak [70]. The Soviet model sanitary-epidemiological system had been very effective in tackling communicable disease in the post-war period but was unable to adapt to the challenge of noncommunicable diseases [71,72]. As in many countries, a career in public health was less enticing than many of the alternatives, thus attracting many of the weakest graduates, a situation exacerbated by undergraduate specialization in the USSR.

Public health functions can, of course, reside in many other settings, within government, academia, and nongovernmental organizations. In many countries these functions were also weak or, in the case of nongovernmental bodies, virtually nonexistent. With a few exceptions, as in Hungary, Czechoslovakia, Poland, and the Baltic Republics, statistical offices confined their activities to the minimum necessary to satisfy the reporting requirements of The World Health Organization (WHO). In some places the academic public health community was somewhat stronger, but these were isolated examples.

There were, however, specific problems in the Soviet Union, where access to ideas developed elsewhere was extremely limited (the Baltic Republics were an exception as they were able to maintain contacts with the west, in the case of Estonia because of a close linguistic affinity with nearby Finland). Thus, Marxist–Leninist teaching was that many of the emerging threats to health were transient, attributable to the transition to communism, and thus expected to resolve spontaneously over time [73]. A rejection of experimental methods, linked with an absence of effective peer-review and an extremely hierarchical academic structure, in which knowledge accumulated only with age, led to many ideas that had no scientific basis and which were often harmful. The use of transfusions to treat undernourished Romanian children is an extreme example, but there are many more. Many are the legacy of a Ukrainian agriculturalist, Trofim Lysenko [74]. He rejected Mendelian ideas, arguing that change in plants arose from adaptation to changing circumstances within a few generations. Although Lysenko was eventually discredited in the 1960s, his views remained widely held for several decades and the academic culture that allowed him to thrive was the same in which many senior Soviet public health scientists were trained, and where voicing a contrary view could easily lead to the gulag, and thus to premature death [75]. While many of the particular beliefs that emerged from this system are now of historical interest, their true legacy is of a culture in which dissent and open debate, especially with those in senior positions, are often strongly discouraged.

A third issue was a lack of clear ownership. No-one was responsible for broadly defined population health. Finally, effective public health interventions often require working across sectors. However the widespread use of highly centralized vertical programmes conspired against collaboration at local level and central government ministries guarded their responsibilities jealously [76,77].

The situation has changed substantially since 1990 but there are still many problems. A review of the Russian language literature on the determinants of trends in health in Russia found little evidence of awareness of relevant research published in western journals or of modern epidemiological methods [78]. Analytic capacity remains weak. Many ministries of health have become even weaker than in the communist period. The sanitary-epidemiological system has remained relatively untouched by the process of reform, partly reflecting the low priority given them by government but also their reluctance to adopt new ideas, in some countries due to widespread corruption among a group that is invested with much discretionary power but low wages and little accountability.

Public health training initiatives

New schools of public health, with staff who have received training abroad teaching modern public health concepts, have emerged in several countries [79]. Some, such as the Hungarian School of Public Health in Debrecen, Hungary, or the Andrija Stamapr School of Public Health, in Zagreb, Croatia, are now well established and use innovative learning methods, combining Masters and Doctoral level training with short courses. There are many examples of innovation, such as the establishment by the Hungarian School of Public Health of a network of sentinel health monitoring stations that provide data for research and teaching, as well as facilitating close links with public health practitioners. The Andrija Stampar School of Public Health runs a successful summer school each year attracting participants from across central and eastern Europe and the former Soviet Union. Elsewhere, several networks of academic centers have developed, such as BRIMHEALTH, established by the Nordic School of Public Health and bringing together centers in the Baltic Republics and

North-Western Russia, or the network of departments established in Russia, which is linked with Hadassah University in Jerusalem, with support from the Russian Soros Foundation and the Israeli government. Several of these centers, such as the Hungarian School and the Moscow Medical Academy, are now participating in major international research programmes.

Unfortunately the situation is less encouraging in some other countries, in particular in the former Soviet Union outside Russia, where there are only a few isolated developments, in countries such as Armenia, Kazakhstan, and Uzbekistan, and generally very little capacity.

The Open Society Institute (OSI) [80], which has provided support to all of these ventures, has recently established a major development programme, involving twinning with western Schools of Public Health and in partnership with the Association of Schools of Public Health in the European Region (ASPHER) [81]. This aims to help established schools to develop further and to support the development of other nascent projects. The new institutions that are emerging will only become effective if they can draw on appropriate, locally relevant evidence on the causes of disease and the appropriate responses. As the preceding sections have shown, the many natural experiments that have taken place in eastern Europe have provided important new insights on the determinants of health and disease. They have, however, also illustrated some of the challenges facing public health researchers in this region.

Conclusions

The challenges to public health in eastern Europe are considerable. Overall levels of health continue to lag well behind those in the west and, in some places are continuing to deteriorate. Old threats, such as tuberculosis, are reappearing and new ones, such as smoking among women and HIV, are emerging for the first time. Some once functioning health care systems are disintegrating. But there are also many examples of success. Death rates from cardiovascular disease are falling rapidly in some countries. Transition-related increases in injury deaths are being brought under control. However, many of these successes owe more to wider societal changes, such as growing prosperity and opening of markets, than to specific public health policies. Unfortunately, the public health infrastructure remains weak in many countries.

Several needs are apparent. One is a greater number of people from a wide range of disciplines trained in modern public health. In some countries newly established schools of public health are already making a substantial contribution to this goal. These individuals need a secure career structure that rewards them sufficiently to ensure their retention and gives them the opportunity to use their newly developed skills to develop and implement the healthy public policies that are noticeable by their absence. These changes will only come about if politicians recognize the need to improve the health of their population, recognizing that progress is possible and necessary. The international community has a role to play in supporting these efforts and the research on which effective policies can be based.

References

[1] McKee M, Healy J, Falkingham J. Health care systems in the Central Asian Republics: An introduction. In: M McKee, J Healy, J Falkingham (eds.). *Health Care in Central Asia.* Buckingham: Open University Press, 2002, pp. 3–11.

[2] Zatonski WA, McMichael AJ, Powles JW. Ecological study of reasons for sharp decline in mortality from ischaemic heart disease in Poland since 1991. *BMJ* 1998; **316**: 1047–51.

[3] Bobak M, Skodova Z, Pisa Z et al. Political changes and trends in cardiovascular risk factors in the Czech Republic, 1985–92. *J Epidemiol Comm Health* 1997; **51**: 272–7.

[4] Nolte E, Shkolnikov V, McKee M. Changing mortality patterns in east and west Germany and Poland: II. Short-term trends during transition and in the 1990s. *J Epidemiol Comm Health* 2000; **54**: 899–906.

[5] Anderson BA, Silver BD. Issues of data quality in assessing mortality trends and levels in the New Independent States. In: *Premature Death in the New Independent States.* Washington DC: National Academy Press, 1997.

[6] Shkolnikov VM, Meslé F, Vallin J. Health crisis in Russia I. Recent trends in life expectancy and causes of death from 1970 to 1993. *Population* 1996; **8**: 123–54.

[7] McKee M, Chenet L. Patterns of health. In: M McKee, J Healy, J Falkingham (eds). *Health Care in Central Asia.* Buckingham: Open University Press, 2002, pp. 57–66.

[8] Badurashvili I, McKee M, Tsuladze G, Meslé F, Vallin J, Shkolnikov V. Where there are no data: What has happened to life expectancy in Georgia since 1990? *Public Health* 2001; **115**: 394–400.

[9] Bozicevic I, Oreskovic S, Stevanovic R et al. What is happening to the health of the Croatian population? *Croatian Med J* 2001; **42**: 601–605.

[10] Checkland P. *Systems Thinking, Systems Practice.* Chichester: Wiley, 1981.

[11] Leon DA. Common threads: underlying components of inequalities in mortality between and within countries. In: D Leon, G Walt (eds.). *Poverty, Inequality and Health.* Oxford: Oxford University Press, 2001, pp. 58–87.

[12] Kuh D, Ben Shlomo Y. *A Life Course Approach to Chronic Disease Epidemiology.* Oxford: Oxford University Press, 1997.

[13] McKee M, Shkolnikov V. Understanding the toll of premature death among men in eastern Europe. *BMJ* 2001; **323**: 1051–5.

[14] Kozintez C, Matusa R, Cazacu A. The changing epidemic of pediatric HIV infection in Romania. *Ann Epidemiol* 2000; **10**: 474–5.

[15] Leon D, Chenet L, Shkolnikov VM et al. Huge variation in Russian mortality rates 1984–1994: Artefact, alcohol, or what? *Lancet* 1997; **350**: 383–8.

[16] Winston FK, Rineer C, Menon R, Baker SP. The carnage wrought by major economic change: Ecological study of traffic related mortality and the reunification of Germany. *BMJ* 1999; **318**: 1647–50.

[17] White S. *Russia Goes Dry*. Cambridge: Cambridge University Press, 1996.

[18] McKee M, Shkolnikov V, Leon DA. Alcohol is implicated in the fluctuations in cardiovascular disease in Russia since the 1980s. *Ann Epidemiol* 2001; **11**: 1–6.

[19] Walberg P, McKee M, Shkolnikov V et al. Economic change, crime, and mortality crisis in Russia: A regional analysis. *BMJ* 1998; **317**: 312–8.

[20] Shkolnikov V, McKee M, Chervyakov VV, Kyrianov NA. Is the link between alcohol and cardiovascular death among young Russian men due to misclassification of acute alcohol intoxication? Evidence from the city of Izhevsk. *J Epidemiol Comm Health* 2002; **56**: 171–4.

[21] Chervyakov VV, Shkolnikov VM, Pridemore WA et al. The changing nature of murder in Russia. *Soc Sci Med* (in press).

[22] McKee M, Zatonski W. How the cardiovascular burden of illness is changing in Eastern Europe. Evidence-based Cardiovascular Medicine 1998; 2: 39–41.

[23] Laks T, Tuomilehto J, Joeste E et al. Alarmingly high occurrence and case fatality of acute coronary heart disease events in Estonia: Results from the Tallinn AMI register 1991–94. *J Intern Med* 1999; 246: 53–60.

[24] Vikhert AM, Tsiplenkova VG, Cherpachenko NM. Alcoholic cardiomyopathy and sudden cardiac death. *J Am Col Card* 1986; 8: 3A–11A.

[25] Perova NV, Oganov RG, Williams DH et al. Association of high-density-lipoprotein cholesterol with mortality and other risk factors for major chronic noncommunicable diseases in samples of US and Russian men. *Ann Epidemiol* 1995; 5: 179–85.

[26] Shakhov YA, Oram JF, Perova NV et al. Comparative study of the activity and composition of HDL3 in Russian and American men. *Arterioscler Thromb* 1993; **13**: 1770–8.

[27] Virchow R. *Phlogose and thrombose in gefassystem. Gessammelte Abhandlungen zur Wissenschaftlichen Medecin*. Staatsdruckerie: Frankfurt, 1856.

[28] West SG. Effect of diet on vascular reactivity: An emerging marker for vascular risk. *Curr Atheroscler Rep* 2001; 3(6): 446–55.

[29] Pomerleau J, McKee M, Robertson A et al. Macronutrient and food intake in the Baltic republics. *Eur J Clin Nutr* 2001; **55**: 200–7.

[30] Bobak M, Brunner E, Miller NJ et al. Could antioxidants play a role in high rates of coronary heart disease in the Czech Republic? *Eur J Clin Nutr* 1998; **52**: 632–6.

[31] Bobak M, McKee M, Rose R, Marmot M. Alcohol consumption in a national sample of the Russian population. *Addiction* 1999; **94**: 857–66.

[32] Britton A, McKee M. The relationship between alcohol and cardiovascular disease in Eastern Europe: explaining the paradox. *J Epidemiol Comm Health* 2000; **54**: 328–32.

[33] McKee M, Britton A. The positive relationship between alcohol and heart disease in eastern Europe: potential physiological mechanisms. *J Roy Soc Med* 1998; **91**: 402–7.

[34] Bobak M, Marmot M. East–West mortality divide and its potential explanations: proposed research agenda. *BMJ* 1996; **312**: 421–5.

[35] Pudule I, Grinberga D, Kadziauskiene K et al. Patterns of smoking in the Baltic Republics. *J Epidemiol Comm Health* 1999; **53**: 277–83.

[36] McKee M, Bobak M, Rose R et al. Patterns of smoking in Russia. *Tobacco Control* 1998; **7**: 22–6.

[37] Zatonski W, Smans M, Tyczynski J et al. Atlas of Cancer Mortality in Central Europe. IARC Scientific Publications No. 134 International Agency for Research on Cancer, Lyon, France, 1996.

[38] Shkolnikov V, McKee M, Leon D, Chenet L. Why is the death rate from lung cancer falling in the Russian Federation? *Eur J Epidemiol* 1999; **15**: 203–6.

[39] Hurt RD. Smoking in Russia: what do Stalin and Western tobacco companies have in common? *Mayo Clin Proc* 1995; **70**: 1007–11.

[40] Bray I, Brennan P, Boffetta P. Projections of alcohol- and tobacco-related cancer mortality in Central Europe. *Int J Cancer* 2000; **87**: 122–8.

[41] Fagerstrom K, Boyle P, Kunze M, Zatonski W. The anti-smoking climate in EU countries and Poland. *Lung Cancer* 2001; **32**: 1–5.

[42] Levi F, Lucchini F, Negri E et al. Cervical cancer mortality in young women in Europe: patterns and trends. *Eur J Cancer* 2000; **36**: 2266–71.

[43] Markina SS, Maksimova NM, Vitek CR et al. Diphtheria in the Russian Federation in the 1990s. *J Infect Dis* 2000; 181 (Suppl 1): S27–34.

[44] Platt L, McKee M. Observations of the management of sexually transmitted diseases in the Russian Federation: a challenge of confidentiality. *Int J STD AIDS* 2000; **11**: 563–67.

[45] Dobson R. AIDS–dramatic surge in ex-Soviet Union, no respite worldwide, new data show. *Bull World Health Organ* 2001; **79**: 78.

[46] Stern V. Sentenced to die. The problem of TB in prisons in Eastern Europe and central Asia. London: International Centre for Prison Studies, Kings College London, 1999.

[47] Farmer PE, Kononets AS, Borisov SE et al. Recrudescent tuberculosis in the Russian Federation. In: PE Farmer, LB Reichman, MD Iseman (eds.).

The Global Impact of Drug Resistant Tuberculosis. Boston MA: Harvard Medical School/ Open Society Institute, 1999.

[48] Stoilova Y, Popivanova N. Epidemiologic studies of leptospiroses in the Plovdiv region of Bulgaria. *Folia Med (Plovdiv)* 1999; **41**: 73–9.

[49] Randolph SE. The shifting landscape of tick-borne zoonoses: tick-borne encephalitis and Lyme borreliosis in Europe. *Philos Trans R Soc Lond B Biol Sci* 2001; **356**: 1045–56.

[50] Leviatan U, Cohen J. Gender differences in life expectancy among kibbutz members. *Soc Sci Med* 1985; **21**: 545–51.

[51] Jedrychowski W, Tobiasz-Adamczyk B, Olma A, Gradzikiewicz P. Survival rates among Seventh day Adventists compared with the general population in Poland. *Scand J Soc Med* 1985; **13**: 49–52.

[52] Chenet L, Leon D, McKee M, Vassin S. Death from alcohol and violence in Moscow: Socio-economic determinants. *Eur J Population* 1998; **14**: 19–37.

[53] Kennedy BP, Kawachi I, Brainerd E. The role of social capital in the Russian mortality crisis. *World Development* 1998; **26**: 2029–43.

[54] Shkolnikov VM, Leon D, Adamets S et al. Educational level and adult mortality in Russia: an analysis of routine data 1979 to 1994. *Soc Sci Med* 1998; **47**: 357–69.

[55] Hajdu P, McKee M, Bojan F. Changes in premature mortality differentials by marital status in Hungary and in England and Wales. *Eur J Publ Health* 1995; **5**: 259–64.

[56] Bobak M, Pikhart H, Hertzman C et al. Socioeconomic factors, perceived control and self-reported health in Russia. A cross-sectional survey. *Soc Sci Med* 1998; **47**: 269–79.

[57] Watson P. Marriage and mortality in eastern Europe. In: C Hertzman, S Kelly, M Bobak (eds). *East–West Life Expectancy Gap in Europe: Environmental and Non-environmental Determinants.* Dordrecht: Kluwer, 1996.

[58] Rose R. Russia as an hour-glass society: a constitution without citizens. *East European Constitutional Review* 1995; **4**: 34–42.

[59] Cockerham WC. Health lifestyles in Russia. *Soc Sci Med* 2000; **51**: 1313–24.

[60] Mackenbach JP, Looman CWN, Kunst AE et al. Post-1950 mortality trends and medical care: gains in life expectancy due to declines in mortality from conditions amenable to medical intervention in The Netherlands. *Soc Sci Med* 1988; **27**: 889–94.

[61] Velkova A, Wolleswinkel-van den Bosch JH, Mackenbach JP. The east–west life expectancy gap: Differences in mortality from conditions amenable to medical intervention. *Int J Epidemiol* 1997; **26**: 75–84.

[62] Goldenberg S. *Pride of Small Nations: The Caucasus and post-Soviet Disorder.* London: Zed, 1994.

[63] Nolte E, Scholz R, Shkolnikov V, McKee M. The contribution of medical care to changing life expectancy in Germany and Poland. *Soc Sci Med* (in press).

[64] Becker N, Boyle P. Decline in mortality from testicular cancer in West
      Germany after reunification. *Lancet* 1997; **350**: 744.

[65] Koupilová I, McKee M, Holčik J. Neonatal mortality in the Czech Republic
      during the transition. *Health Policy* 1998; **46**: 43–52.

[66] Nolte E, Hort A, Koupilová I, McKee M. Trends in neonatal and postneonatal
      mortality in the eastern and western parts of Germany after unification.
      J Epidemiol Comm Health 2000; **54**: 84–90.

[67] Telishevska M, Chenet L, McKee M. Towards an understanding of the high
      death rate among young people with diabetes in Ukraine. *Diab Med* 2001;
      18: 3–9.

[68] McKee M, Zwi A, Koupilová I et al. Health policy-making in central and
      eastern Europe: lessons from the inaction on injuries? *Health Policy Planning*
      2000; **15**: 263–9.

[69] Chenet L, McKee M, Fulop N et al. Changing life expectancy in central
      Europe: is there a single reason? *J Publ Health Med* 1996; **18**: 329–36.

[70] McKee M, Bojan F, Normand C, on behalf of the TEMPUS consortium for a
      new public health in Hungary. A new programme for public health training
      in Hungary. *Eur J Publ Health* 1993; **3**: 58–63.

[71] McKee M, Bojan F. In: J Figueras et al. (eds.). *Reforming Public Health
      Services Critical Challenges for Health Care Reform*. Open University Press,
      1998, pp. 135–54.

[72] Bojan F, McKee M, Ostbye T. Status and priorities of public health in
      Hungary. Zeitschrift für Gesundheitswissenschaften 1994; (Suppl 1): 48–55.

[73] Deacon B. Medical care and health under state socialism. *Int J Health Serv*
      1984; **14**: 453–80.

[74] Joravsky D. *The Lysenko Affair*. Chicago: Univ Chicago Press, 1970.

[75] Soyfer VN. The consequences of political dictatorship for Russian science.
      Nat Rev Genet 2001; **2**: 723–9.

[76] Gorbachev M. *Memoirs*. London: Doubleday, 1996.

[77] Varvasovszky Z, McKee M. An analysis of alcohol policy in Hungary. Who is
      in charge? *Addiction* 1998; **93**: 1815–27.

[78] Tkatchenko E, McKee M, Tsouros AD. Public health in Russia: the view from
      the inside. *Health Policy Planning* 2000; **15**: 164–9.

[79] McKee M, Bojan F, White M, Ostbye T. Development of public health
      training in Hungary—an exercise in international co-operation. *J Publ
      Health Med* 1995; **17**: 438–44.

[80] http://www.soros.org/.

[81] http://www.ensp.fr/aspher/.

Chapter 6

Public health in North America

F Douglas Scutchfield and John M Last

The United States of America and Canada share the North American land mass, indigenous societies that were disrupted and virtually destroyed by European colonists, and closely intertwined economies and trade, which have been enhanced by the North America Free Trade Agreement. Ideas, particularly in health, health care, and public health flow freely across the border. As a consequence of these links, public health shares many common features in the two countries, although the two nations differ in their methods of payment for personal and hospital medical care.

In the final four decades of the twentieth century, Canadian leadership in public health and preventive medicine influenced the practice, policies, and research priorities in, and beyond, both nations. In 1974, the Government of Canada published a landmark document, *A New Perspective on the Health of Canadians*, known as the Lalonde Report [1] signed by the Minister of Health, Marc Lalonde. The report criticized the conventional view that investment in care of the sick was the highest priority; it pointed out that the predominant health problems were attributable to environmental factors, behavior ("lifestyle"), or aberrations of human biology, and that these, along with provision of health care—including health-promotion—were the real priorities. Lalonde advocated an approach to health improvement based largely on health promotion and disease prevention, a notion that found favor outside Canada. These ideas contributed to the rise of the health promotion movement, the "healthy cities, healthy communities" initiatives that led to close collaboration between Canada and the European regional office of World Health Organization (WHO), and to the first WHO conference on health promotion in Ottawa in 1984 and the Ottawa Charter on Health Promotion [2]. The Lalonde Report was also an antecedent to the initial 1979 US Surgeon General's Report on Health Promotion and Disease Prevention, to which we will refer later [3].

Another example of Canadian leadership in public health and preventive medicine was the establishment in the mid-1970s of the Task Force on the Periodic Health Examination. The task force reviewed and evaluated a great many available interventions aimed at promoting good health and the early detection of serious diseases such as cancer and cardiovascular diseases [4,5]. The Canadian leadership in clinical preventive medicine was followed closely in the United States, and the Canadian and US Task Forces on preventive services have worked in close collaboration. Both have adopted the evidence-based approach originally developed in Canada [4] and have made similar recommendations.

Health status in North America

Overall both countries have similar health problems, with the leading causes of death being cancer, heart disease, and stroke and the major underlying risk factors being the same. In addition, both countries have substantial inequalities in health status particularly among African Americans and Native Americans. Vital and health statistics do not usually list indicators separately or in sufficient detail to reveal the unfavorable experience of Native Americans (known as First Nations in Canada). However, there is abundant information from specialized studies and reports, all painting a consistent picture.

Infant, perinatal and child mortality rates are higher and life expectancy is lower among both African Americans and Native Americans than in the "whites" (Europeans) in both the Canadian and American general population. Substance abuse, alcohol addiction, suicide—especially among young males—sexually transmitted diseases, and HIV/AIDS, all have higher prevalence rates in native Americans, as do diabetes and arthritis. Among African Americans, the health inequalities reflect in part the occupational and economic differences. Poorer educational opportunities, higher unemployment, and ghettoized living conditions tend to encourage violent crime, including homicide, among young black males. In middle age the common causes of death—cardiovascular disease, stroke, and some cancers (notably breast cancer and prostate cancer) and diabetes all hit African Americans harder than white Americans. Moreover, the provision of all forms of health care, ranging from primary preventive services to specialized tertiary hospital care, is more often deficient in communities that serve African Americans than those serving whites. These public health problems are the same as those found in similar population groups in other parts of the world where European colonization marginalized indigenous people and destroyed their pre-colonial habitat and culture. In the United States, the health problems of those who are descended from African immigrants brought unwillingly to America as slaves are generally more severe than those of all but the most disadvantaged indigenous peoples. Public health services have so far failed to find a satisfactory solution to this complex cluster of problems [6].

Income inequalities are less striking in Canada than in the United States, there is a more secure social safety net, and social cohesiveness is overall probably stronger in Canada than in the United States. These factors contribute to the overall more favorable health experience of Canada compared to the United States as measured by life expectancy, infant mortality, and disability-adjusted life years lost; on all of these indicators, Canada has consistently out-performed the United States. Throughout most of the 1990s, Canada was the first among the world's nations on the Human Development Index, and consistently ranks among the first three countries. The extent, if any, to which public health services contribute to this favorable health profile is debatable. The benefits of health protection measures such as environmental sanitation and communicable disease control are well known and abundantly confirmed by statistical indicators (although in many rural communities there are deficiencies that lead to occasional outbreaks of diarrheal diseases). However, the contribution to health improvement of expenditure and professional expertise devoted to health promotion remain largely uncertain; no systematic evaluations have been done either in the United States or in Canada.

The organization of public health services

We use as an organizing structure for this chapter the 1988 US Institute of Medicine (IOM) Report, The Future of Public Health [7]. The IOM report made several contributions to the work of public health, notably regarding the responsibilities of various levels of government for public health functions. It also made recommendations for the organization of public health services and programs at federal, state (in Canada, provincial), and local levels. The report defined public health's mission as "assuring conditions in which people can be healthy". The report then focused on the official public health agencies at the local, state, and federal level.

Public health functions

The report recommended that the functions that all public health agencies should be performing are assessment, policy development, and assurance. The report defines assessment as: ". . . regularly and systematically collect, assemble, analyze and make available information on the health of the community, including statistics on health status, community health needs, and epidemiological and other studies of health problems".[7] In terms of policy development, the Report suggests that every public agency should: "... serve the public's interest in the development of comprehensive public health policies by promoting the use of the scientific knowledge base in decision-making about public health and by leading in developing public health policy".[7] By assurance the report meant: "... assure their constituents that services necessary to achieve agreed upon goals are provided, either by encouraging actions by other entities (private or public sector), by requiring such action through regulation, or by providing services directly".[7]

Unfortunately, this trilogy of public health functions is difficult to explain to many stakeholders, notably policy makers and legislators. During the US health system reform debate of the early 1990s, it was important to communicate to stakeholders the contribution to health improvement of public health and the work of health departments. In that context, a group of public health stakeholders came together to further refine and develop a broader group of public health essential functions/services that would more easily communicate what public health is and does. This led to the creation of a list of ten essential public health functions:

(1) monitor health status to identify community health problems;

(2) diagnose and investigate health problems and health hazards in the community;

(3) inform, educate, and empower people about health issues;

(4) mobilize community partnerships to identify and solve health problems;

(5) develop policies and plans that support individual and community health efforts;

(6) enforce laws and regulations that protect health and ensure safety;

(7) link people to needed personal health services and assure the provision of health care when otherwise unavailable;

(8) assure a competent public health care workforce;

(9) evaluate effectiveness, accessibility, and quality of personal and population-based health services;

(10) research for new insights and innovative solutions to health problems [8].

These essential public health functions have become a beginning point for a number of public health activities in the United States, such as the

National Public Health Performance Measures Program, the development of competencies for public health professionals, and the development of a research agenda in public health.

Provision of basic health care services

The role of the public health agency in providing medical care is important enough for a brief digression. In the United States substantial debate continues about whether the public health agency has a duty and responsibility to provide illness care to those unable to afford it or with limited access to health care services. In 1966, the US federal government passed the Medicaid Act, a health insurance plan for some poor individuals. In many cases, public health agencies began to provide direct patient care services to uninsured and to medicaid patients. The medicaid funding stream became an important source of revenue for public health agencies. However, with an increase in numbers of physicians and state government efforts to move medicaid patients in to the main stream of medical care, this source of funding for local health departments has either decreased or disappeared entirely. This has created difficulties for those health departments who would like to assume a direct patient care role. They no longer have that funding stream to support this function. In addition, some health departments were using medicaid to subsidize direct patient care to uninsured individuals. In Canada the comprehensive national health insurance program ensures that this problem does not arise for public health services.

Approximately 14 percent of the US population, or forty-four million individuals, do not have any health insurance [9]. An issue of social justice is how to assure that these people receive needed medical care. In the United States a group of organizations and agencies, characterized as the "safety network", assume responsibility for caring for these people. This includes public hospitals, federally funded community health centers, not-for-profit hospitals and their emergency rooms. The issue is should the safety net also include the health department? There is no question that the public health agency should be providing clinical preventive services, such as immunizations, but should the health department also provide primary health care? Critics of the notion of public health agencies providing medical care point out it can divert resources from the core public health services that must be provided to the entire community population. This debate continues without a clear-cut answer. The obvious solution is to provide health insurance to the entire US population, so that they may use the medical care system for those needs and provide adequate funding for public health agencies for them to provide needed population-based services. That is an easily articulated vision, but given the political nature of the provision of health care in the United States, not easy to implement.

In this regard Canada is far ahead of the United States. Canada passed in 1967 a comprehensive, universal, publicly administered medical and hospital insurance plan that covers the entire population; the diversion of public health energy for indigent care is not an issue in Canada.

Organization and responsibilities of US public health agencies

The primary responsibility for public health in the United States rests at the state level. The US Constitution does not mention health as a federal responsibility and according to other provisions in the Constitution, everything not delegated to the federal government remains a state responsibility; thus, states have the "police power" to assure the health of the population. The United States adopted the English statutory and common law that recognizes the responsibility of the state to protect the health and safety of its citizen's [10].

While the state has this responsibility, in most cases it delegates the responsibility and authority to a governmental entity closer to the people; localities have been given, usually by state statute, specific duties and activities that they are required by state action to undertake. In most cases, some proportion of the state's funding flows to the locality to accomplish those delegated tasks. Essentially similar organizational arrangements prevail in Canada, where funding for public health services is provided partly by each level of revenue-generation, i.e. federal, provincial, and local.

The US federal government is active in health as the result of two major responsibilities that it has under the Constitution: the right to regulate interstate commerce and the right to tax and spend. Pundits quip that in the United States, the locals have the problem, the state has the authority, and the federal government has the money.

Given this context, let's examine, using the framework of the Future of Public Health, recommendations about the character and nature of public health at the federal state and local level.

The federal government

The IOM report defines the federal government's obligations in public health as:

(1) support of knowledge development and dissemination through data gathering, research, and information exchange;

(2) establishment of nationwide health objectives and priorities, and stimulation of debate on interstate and national public health issues;

(3) provision of technical assistance to help states determine their own objectives and to carry out action on national and regional objectives;

(4) provision of funds to strengthen state capacity for services, especially to achieve an adequate minimum capacity, and to achieve national objectives;

(5) assurance of actions and services that are in the public interest of the entire nation such as control of AIDS and similar communicable diseases, interstate environmental actions, and food and drug inspection [7].

It is beyond the scope of this chapter to develop, in detail, each of these obligations for each level of government. Nevertheless, it is useful to consider several of these obligations.

Establishing national objectives

One of the federal government's most effective efforts is that of establishing national goals and objectives. The Lalonde Report, in Canada, gave rise to a similar effort in the United States. The first document in a series of relevant publications, flowing from the Lalonde Report, was Healthy People, The Surgeon General's Report on Health Promotion and Disease Prevention, published in 1979 [3]. This document established a series of age related goals for mortality and, in the case of the elderly, morbidity, to be achieved by the year 1990 and the priority program areas, which, if appropriately implemented, would allow these targets to be achieved. Following this publication, the US Public Health Services convened a group that developed, for the Surgeon General's priority program areas, specific objectives to be achieved by the year 1990. This resulted in the creation of a second document, Health Promotion Disease Prevention: Objectives for the Nation [11].

Canada's health goals and targets were discussed by provincial task forces rather than at federal (national) level, because health is a provincial responsibility. The result was a patchwork quilt of recommendations that, because of political and philosophical differences and changes in some provincial governments, were largely ineffectual [12]. The initiative passed back to the federal government with the establishment of the National Forum on Health in 1993. This was a nationwide assembly of experts in all fields related to health policy (medicine and health sciences, economics, ethics, law, consumer groups, etc.). The National Forum on Health reported in 1997 directly to the Prime Minister [13] and made recommendations on many aspects of current health problems of Canadians, for example, needs of vulnerable groups, realignment of hospital-based specialist services, and community oriented primary care and preventive services, but left open the issue of future funding. In 2002 this issue is being explored further. Alberta, which has a far-right conservative administration, is actively developing a wide range of private services while undermining the public basis of medical care.

The American efforts provided an opportunity to mobilize all levels of government and non-governmental organizations and agencies to focus on some common themes that had the potential to improve health status. In fact, many states developed state level companion documents consistent with national objectives. This objective setting proved successful and in the late 1980s a second effort was launched to develop an expanded set of objectives to be achieved by the year 2000. This process resulted in Healthy People 2000 [14]. Again, this met with general acceptance and a similar process was undertaken in the late 1990s resulting in Healthy People 2010 [15]. While the iteration of this activity has generally met with wide approval, it does have its critics who have commented on the number and diversity of objectives and their seeming lack of focus [16].

Data collection and dissemination

Both the state and federal governments, according to the IOM report, have responsibility in this area and collaborate in this effort. In many cases the federal government will provide funding to states to collect data, which is then passed on to the federal level. A good illustration is the Behavioral Risk Factor Surveillance System. The federal government provides funding to states to undertake a random digit dialing survey of adults in the state to ascertain risk factors for disease. These data are reported to the federal government that compiles national data that can be used for benchmarks for each state to determine progress and to make appropriate program modifications to address areas where they are falling short [17]. All states compile and report vital events such as births and deaths. In addition, information on certain diseases, usually communicable diseases, are compiled by the state and reported to the federal government. States, may and frequently do, add extra diseases to the reporting system for which there may be local interest.

States

The IOM report defines the obligations of the state in the public health mission as:

* assessment of health needs based on statewide data collection;
* assurance of an adequate statutory base for health activities in the state;

- establishment of statewide health objectives, delegating power to localities as appropriate and holding them accountable;
- assurance of appropriate statewide effort to develop and maintain essential personal, educational, and environmental health services; provision of access to necessary services; and solution of problems inimical to health;
- guarantee of a minimum set of essential health services;
- support of local service capacity, especially when disparities in local ability to raise revenue and/or administer programs requiring subsidies, technical assistance, or direct action by the state to achieve adequate service levels [7].

Statutory base for public health

The states have primary responsibility for public health, as previously discussed. They have the police power to protect the health of their citizens. In order to appropriately discharge that authority, they need a legal base on which to operate. The state has the responsibility to examine their laws to assure that there is clear understanding of the scope and nature of authority to officials and the boards that have public health oversight. They should appropriately delineate the relationship between state and local government, recognizing that the authority local health departments have is derived from the authority of the state; many of the public health statues were written in an earlier time and modern public health procedures have often outstripped those statues.

State local relations

As described above, the authority of the local health departments derives from the primary authority of the state. The state serves, as it were, as the parent of local health departments; the state has responsibility to assist the local health department in its efforts. That assistance may take many forms, financial, knowledge, and direction. Generally, local health departments derive their budgets from several sources: federal money (generally given to the state and "passed through" to localities), state general fund money, fees charged for services rendered generally either for direct patient care or for licensing/inspection fees, and local tax revenue. There is a mix of relationships of funding and organization with state/local relations. In some cases there is not a local health department and all local health employees and the locality's budget are part of the state health department. In other cases, a minor portion of the local health department's budget is provided by the state. In some states, not every local jurisdiction has a local health department and the state must assume responsibility to provide those services. In some cases the jurisdiction may be so small that the budget it can generate from any source is inadequate to assure a minimum level of services; in this case the state must step in to assure adequate resources to assure needed services.

States must hold localities accountable for assuring that essential public health services are provided. While this has been problematic in the past, new activities are underway to develop methods for accountability. The Nation Public Health Performance Standards Program is working to create tools for state and local health units and local governing boards to ascertain their performance in achieving the core/essential services described above [18]. There is no licensure or certification of health departments, with minor exception, although this national program has the potential to change this unsatisfactory situation. In addition, many jurisdictions do not have personnel with adequate knowledge to deal with some major public health issues. For example, it would be unusual for a small local health department to have a trained epidemiologist or a laboratory. In these circumstances the state must provide this expertise.

Local health departments

The IOM report suggests the following functions for local health departments:

(1) assessment, monitoring, and surveillance of local health problems and needs and of resources for dealing with them;

(2) policy development and leadership that foster local involvement and a sense of ownership, that emphasize local needs, and that advocate equitable distribution of public resources and complementary private activities commensurate with community needs;

(3) assurance that high-quality services, including personal health services, needed for the protection of public health in the community are available and accessible for all persons; that the community receives proper consideration in the allocation of federal and state as well as local resources for public health; and that the community is informed about how to obtain public health, including personal health services, or how to comply with public health requirements [7].

Canadian organization for the delivery of public health services

Canada resembles the United States in having a division of roles and responsibilities between federal, provincial, and local levels of jurisdiction.

Under the Canadian Constitution, both health and education are provincial responsibilities. Federal–provincial rivalries and differing political philosophies among the levels of government sometimes impair smooth working relationships—a situation familiar also in the United States. The Canada Health Act of 1967 enabled the establishment of the universal comprehensive medical and hospital insurance program and was unusual in demonstrating harmony at all levels of government; generally there are smooth working relationships also in public health services at the three levels of government.

Problems and issues in North America's public health services

A review was completed in 1989 on the implementation of the IOM report's state recommendations, and repeated in 1997, with a companion report on local health departments. Both reported modest improvements in the administrative recommendations issued by the IOM [19,20]. However, there continued to be erosion of resources provided to health departments in the United States, as reflected in the data on revenue to local health departments collected by the National Association of City and County Health Officials (NACCHO) [21]. The increasing reliance of health departments on patient care funding reduced their capacity to provide core public health functions.

In addition, since the 1960s attention has focused on issues of assess to care for all individuals. While this is an appropriate goal, given limited resources, these federal and state health dollars were frequently diverted from money which could, and may previously, have gone to support public health. Thus, through the latter half of the last century there has been an erosion in the ability of the health department to carry out the population based services for the entire population for which they are responsible, as documented by the continued data surveillance of local health department revenues by NACCHO [21]. This problem is further compounded by the proclivity to approach health problems on a categorical basis, with no concern for the underlying resources that must exist to provide categorical services. There has been little attention paid to the infrastructure of public health. There is a pattern of inadequate capital expenditure on plant and equipment, and insufficient effort devoted to recruitment and training of qualified staff in such disciplines as health inspection, nutrition, and social work oriented to problems peculiar to public health. Salary levels are generally not competitive and attrition rates are high, so many public health departments are chronically short-staffed.

In Canada in the 1990s, conservative, tax-cutting provincial governments were at odds with the federal government. Ontario, the most populous and richest province of Canada, elected a conservative government whose tax-cutting policies led to serious erosion of environmental health protective measures and were the probable cause of several serious outbreaks of water-borne *E. Coli* 0157 infection [22]. A recent and unpublished report indicates that Canada's public health infrastructure may be overwhelmed if it faces more than one major public health crises at once. The system is said to be "on the ropes", that is in a fragile and vulnerable state with inadequate human and technical resources and the situation is getting worse, not better [23].

The functions, and the roles and responsibilities of Canadian staff at federal, provincial, and local levels closely resemble their US counterparts, and generally there are close collegial working relationships across the border so in some ways the systems in the two nations work almost as one. Exceptions, for instance in food safety standards and permissible exposure limits to toxic substances, seldom cause problems. Public health officials recognize that public health problems such as outbreaks of communicable diseases do not end at national borders.

The future

Public health agencies are changing rapidly against a backdrop of rapid national change. Several trends will influence the public health of the future and how services are provided. The development of a so called information society has profound implications for the role of the health department as a major node on the information highway designed to collect, analyze, and disseminate information, not only to professionals but to the public as a whole.

The events of 11 September 2001 and the subsequent experience with anthrax demonstrated the profound impact of an eroded public health infrastructure as we discussed above. It is likely that these events will result in major efforts to rebuild that public health infrastructure, focused on epidemiology and surveillance for both communicable and noncommunicable diseases, workforce development, communication and information technology, and laboratory capacity. It is incumbent on those in public health to ensure that resources coming to public health are used wisely to reinvigorate the public health infrastructure that can be used for any public health issue. The anthrax scare in the autumn of 2001 strengthened the already-strong collaborative bond between the United States and Canada in epidemiological surveillance.

Major changes are continuing in the way medicine, the companion discipline to public health, is practiced which will in turn profoundly effect the delivery of public health services. Modern medical advances such as the sequencing of the genome is an illustration of these developments. Not only scientific advances, but also the way in which health care is funded will also influence the role and responsibility of public health, for example in the delivery of primary care. The globalization of health risks and the emergence or reemergence of diseases, such as West Nile fever, will influence the public health scene of the future. The rise of teen pregnancy and violence, domestic violence, alcohol, and drug abuse are all issues that will require a new way of thinking. The national illicit drug abuse policies of both Canada and the United States have manifestly failed; Canada is nearer than the United States to acknowledging this reality. There are serious discussions about decriminalizing marijuana, which is already legally available on prescription for certain medical conditions; drug abuse is a health problem that will never be conducive to control by police action. These challenges will require public health practitioners to move beyond the traditional knowledge base and may represent an opportunity for the beginning of the third public health revolution [24].

Although the United States and Canada share many social, cultural, and economic characteristics, there are some subtle and important differences in their political systems and philosophical and ideological orientation. These differences are summarized in the catch phrases "Life, liberty and the pursuit of happiness" in the United States, in contrast to the Canadian "Peace, order and good government". Many Americans perceive government as an adversary that, unless they are vigilant, might deprive them of inalienable rights, such as the right to bear arms. Many Canadians, on the other hand, perceive government as the agency that can best help them in times of need. This probably accounts for profoundly different national attitudes toward comprehensive tax-supported personal health care and hospital services, and toward the state's paternalist (interventionist) role in public health services. (It is also reflected in the markedly lower rates of gun ownership, and firearm-related death rates from homicide, suicide, and accidental deaths, that are less than a tenth of those in the United States.) Canadians expect their governments—federal, provincial, and local—to provide and maintain efficient and effective public health services, and get very upset when health protection measures break down as they have done several times in recent years when provincial governments elected on a tax-cutting platform have dismantled existing public health services. Governments that do this can expect to be defeated at the next election. In the United States, on the other hand, many people look to the private sector for solutions to public health problems such as contamination of municipal water supplies, and seem more interested in seeking remedies through litigation after the fact in the courts, rather than through health-protective legislation and regulation.

The United States and Canada have in common a problem shared by many other nations: most of the time, public health services are taken for granted. They are rarely accorded the budgetary priority they need and are regarded as less important, and certainly less glamorous, than high technology surgical and intensive care medical services. Ironically, these expensive aspects of medical care might need less lavish financial support if public health services received their fair share. Only rarely do elected political leaders recognize the importance of maintaining and strengthening public health services, usually when a major crisis occurs, such as a life-threatening epidemic of a communicable disease. If the malicious terrorism of biological war, the anthrax cases that were deliberately spread through the US postal service in 2001, leads to an infusion of funds into federal, state, provincial, and local public health services, and some upgrading of their infrastructure, then it could turn out to be an ill wind that has blown a little good after all.

References

[1] Ottawa. Government of Canada. Lalonde Report: A New Perspective on the Health of Canadians. Ottawa: Government of Canada, 1974.

[2] World Health Organization. A Charter for health promotion (the Ottawa Charter). *Can J Public Health* 1986; 77: 425–30.

[3] US Dept of Health. Education and Welfare. Health People: Surgeon General's Report on Health Promotion and Disease Prevention. Washington, DC: US Dept of Health, Education and Welfare, 1979. PHS publication 79-55071.

[4] Canadian Task Force on the Periodic Health Examination. Periodic versus annual health examination. *Can Med Assoc J* 1979; 121 (Suppl): 1–45.

[5] Ottawa. Ministry of Supply and Services. The Canadian Guide to Clinical Preventive Services. Ottawa. Ministry of Supply and Services, 1994.

[6] Young TK. *The Health of Native Americans*. New York: Oxford University Press, 1994.

[7] Institute of Medicine, Committee for the Study of the Future of Public Health. *The Future of Public Health*. Washington, DC: National Academy Press, 1988.

[8] Harrell J, Baker E. *The Essential Services of Public Health*. Washington, DC: American Public Health Association, 1997.

[9] US Dept of Health and Human Services. Health, United States. Washington, DC: US Dept of Health and Human Services, 1999, PHS 99-1232.

[10] Richards EP, Rathbun KC. The legal basis for public health. In: FD Scutchfield, CW Keck (eds). *Principles of Public Health Practice.* New York: Delmar Publishing, 1997, p. 43.

[11] US Dept of Health and Human Services. Promoting Health/Preventing Disease: Year 2000 Objectives for the Nation. Washington, DC: US Dept of Health and Human Services, 1980.

[12] Spasoff, RA. Health for All Ontario; Report of the Panel on Health Goals for Ontario, Toronto. Ontario: Ministry of Health, 1987.

[13] Ottawa. Department of Public Works and Government Services. Canada Health Action—Building on the Legacy. Final Report of the National Forum on Health. Ottawa: Department of Public Works and Government Services, 1997.

[14] US Dept of Health and Human Services. Healthy People 2000: National Health Promotion and Disease Prevention Objectives. Washington, DC: US Dept of Health and Human Services, 1990. PHS publication 91–50212.

[15] US Department of Health and Human Services. Healthy People 2010. Washington, DC: US Dept of Health and Human Services, 2000. www.health.gov/healthypeople/.

[16] Davis RM. Healthy People 2010: Objectives for the United States: Impressive, but unwieldy. *BMJ* 2000; **320**: 818–19.

[17] Harris JR, McQueen DV, Koplan JP. Chronic disease control. In: FD Scutchfield, CW Keck (eds.). *Principles of Public Health Practice.* New York: Delmar Publishing, 1997, pp. 216–17.

[18] Halverson PK. Performance measurement and performance standards: old wine in new bottles. *J Public Health Manag Pract* 2000; **6**: vi–x.

[19] Scutchfield FD, Hiltabiddle SE, Rawding N et al. Compliance with the recommendations of the Institute of Medicine report: The Future of Public Health: a survey of local health departments. *J Public Health Policy* 1997; **18**: 155–66.

[20] Scutchfield FD, Beversdorf CA, Hiltabiddle SE et al. A survey of state health department compliance with the recommendations of the Institute of Medicine report: The Future of Public Health. *J Public Health Policy* 1997; **18**: 13–29.

[21] National Association of County and City Health Officials. (2001) MAPP Project, available at http://nacchoweb.naccho.org/MAPP_Home.asp.

[22] Walkerton. Ontario outbreak of E Coli 0157: Auld H: The historical significance of rainfall in the Walkerton area during May 2000. Testimony at the Walkerton Inquiry, 15 January 2001.

[23] Editorial. Public health on the ropes. *Can Med Assoc J* 2002; **166**: 1245.

[24] Scutchfield FD, Hartman K. A new preventive medicine for a new millennium. *Aviation, Space & Environmental Medicine* 1996; **67**: 369–75.

Chapter 7

Public health in Latin America

José Noronha, Henri Jouval Jr. and
Cristiani Machado

Introduction

Latin American countries faced significant economic, social and political
changes during the 1990s. The countries were strongly influenced by both
economic globalization and their marginal role in the new global economic
and power arrangements. There were many positives changes in the political sphere, especially with democracy being expanded and consolidated.
However, the expectations of accelerated economic growth and improvements of the social conditions and reduction of inequalities after the
intense slowdown of the 1980s (the "lost decade") remained unachieved.
Economic liberalization enforced throughout the world led to many
adverse changes in the region. Economic growth was lower for most countries in the 1990s as shown in Fig. 7.1 which compares the average annual
growth rate between the 1945–80 and 1990–99 periods for some Latin
American countries [1]. The correction of primary fiscal imbalances and
the control of inflation were not sufficient to promote growth. External
dependency deepened and productivity remained low. External and internal indebtedness increased in the region. Latin America and Caribbean
gross disbursed external debt increased from US$484 billion 1992 to 737
billion in 2000 [2]. In brief, "Globalization has yet to bear its fruits. Currently,
it reproduces longstanding asymmetries and creates new ones, reflecting
the contrast between the rapid internationalization of a few markets and
the absence of a complete, less-biased world agenda". [3]

The slow pace and volatility of economic growth did not reduce either
the number of poor people living in the region nor the inequalities between
and within countries in the region. Great inequalities are the trademark of
the subcontinent. In 1999, 35 percent of Latin America's households were

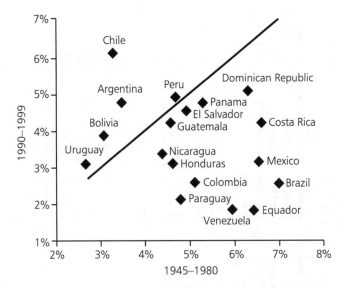

Fig. 7.1 Latin America: Average growth of gross domestic product, 1945–80 and 1990–99
Source: ECLAC, based on official figures.

considered poor and 14 percent were extremely poor or indigent [4]. Compared to the 1980 figures, the number of poor households slightly increased from 35 percent and the number of indigent slightly decreased from 15.0 percent. However the absolute number of people increased in both groups: from twenty-four to forty-one million living in poor households, and from ten to sixteen million in indigent households. The richest 10 percent of the population has more than 30 percent of total income in all countries in Latin America except Costa Rica and Uruguay. The share of total income of the poorest 40 percent is very small, between 9 and 12 percent, with the exception of Uruguay.

Health conditions [5,6]

The Region of the America is divided by the Pan American Health Organization (PAHO) into subregions to allow comparisons between country groups and includes the following subregions: North America; Latin America, comprising the Andean Area, Brazil, Central American Isthmus, Latin Caribbean, Mexico, and the Southern Cone; and the Non-Latin Caribbean. A summary of population indicators is presented in Table 7.1.

Table 7.1 America's basic population indicators 2000: selected indicators by PAHO subregion

Subregion	Total population (millions) 2000	Annual population growth rate (%) 1995–2000	Urban population (%) 2000	Total fertility rate (per woman) 1995–2000	Infant mortality (per 1000 live births) 1995–2000	Life expectancy at birth (years) 1995–2000	Literate population (%) 1998
The Americas	823.2	1.3	76.0	2.4	24.8	72.4	92
North America	308.6	0.8	77.2	1.9	7.0	76.9	99
Latin America & The Caribbean	514.7	1.5	75.3	2.7	35.5	69.8	87
Latin America	506.8	1.5	75.6	2.7	35.7	69.7	87
Mexico	98.9	1.6	74.4	2.8	31.0	72.5	91
Central American Isthmus	36.6	2.5	48.3	3.9	36.0	69.7	75
Latin Caribbean	31.4	1.2	63.4	2.7	45.0	68.3	80
Brazil	169.2	1.2	81.3	2.2	42.0	67.1	85
Andean Area	109.7	1.8	75.0	3.0	35.0	69.7	90
Southern Cone	61.0	1.4	85.3	2.7	22.0	73.3	96
Non-Latin Caribbean	7.9	1.0	58.9	2.3	22.0	72.6	91

Source: PAHO (2000).

The overall population in the Region was estimated at nearly 800 million in 1998, nearly 14 percent of the world's population, and has increased by 25 percent since 1980. Around 37 percent of the population resides in North America, while another third can be found in Brazil and Mexico. The remaining third is scattered among the other forty-three countries and territories in the Region.

The annual population growth rate decreased in the Americas from an estimated average of 1.6 percent in 1980–85 to 1.3 percent in 1995–2000. The subregions with the slowest population increase were North America (0.8 percent) and the Non-Latin Caribbean (1.0 percent). Brazil, Mexico and the Andean Area had an important decrease in their population growth rate, between 22 and 27 percent. In contrast with other subregions, the growth rate in Central America increased slightly, from 2.4 to 2.5 percent during the same period.

Geographical trends in population distribution show higher growth in urban areas and lower growth in rural areas. However, there has been an important change in the concentration of people in metropolitan areas where population growth has slowed. This phenomenon implies that mid-sized cities that can still respond to new demands will grow more rapidly and the excessive growth pressure on the Region's major cities will abate.

Over recent decades infant mortality in the Americas has decreased by around one-third, from an estimated 36.9 deaths per 1000 live births in 1980–85 to 24.8 per 1000 in 1995–2000. Although their infant mortality rates are still higher than the 1980–85 average, the largest gains occurred in Central America (45 percent reduction), Brazil (34 percent reduction) and the Latin Caribbean (30 percent reduction).

Life expectancy at birth has increased in the Americas at an average of 3.2 years, from an estimated 69.2 years in 1980–85 to 72.4 years in 1995– 2000. North America reached the highest levels of life expectancy at birth, 76.9 years in the 1995–2000 period. In contrast, Brazil, the Latin Caribbean, Central America and the Andean Area are still lagging behind the other subregions by several years, although they have experienced increases of between three and eight years [7].

Save for rare exceptions, mortality indicators have improved over the past seven five-year periods for all age groups in every country in the Americas. However, there are large disparities among and within the countries. These disparities become obvious when differential mortality rates by age group and cause of death are compared among those countries presenting a similar economic development level, as determined by per capita income adjusted by their currency's purchasing power.

When countries were grouped in five levels of economic development the infant mortality, for example, showed a sustained downward trend in all the countries and territories of the Americas. During the last fifty years, this trend has represented, in general, a threefold reduction in the infant mortality rate. The dispersion of this indicator—given by the interquartile range—is being reduced progressively within every group of economic income, which suggests an increase in the homogeneity between groups, i.e., a reduction of the inequalities in the risk of dying in infancy within each group. By contrast, the presence of inequalities in infant mortality among the groups of similar income persists in time; for example, the ratio of the median values of infant mortality rate between the two extreme income groups of countries has remained constant during the last three 5-year periods: 6.3 (72.5/11.5), 6.1 (60.5/10.0) and 6.1 (49.0/8.0) [8].

Injury, a major cause of death in the Region, is responsible for between 7 and 25 percent of all deaths, and is a growing problem, reaching epidemic proportions in some countries. In 1998 among America's low and middle income countries (basically Latin America) interpersonal violence and road-traffic injuries ranked fifth and sixth as causes of death, and fifth and third as causes of burden of disease for both sexes. These conditions were the two leading causes of death for the 15–44 age group [9].

Great progress has been made in the struggle against childhood diseases in the countries of the Region. Poliomyelitis was eradicated in 1991, advances have been made in the eradication of measles and neonatal tetanus, the number of episodes of acute diarrhoeal disease has decreased, and significant reductions in mortality from intestinal infectious diseases and acute respiratory infections have occurred. Despite this progress, however, diarrhoeal diseases, acute respiratory infections, and malnutrition remain the leading causes of death in the population under five years of age in most of the medium- and lower-income countries of the Region.

The incidence of AIDS continues to rise in the Region but at a slower rate than in Africa, Asia, and Eastern Europe. All countries now have national programs and surveillance systems. Massive research efforts have resulted in promising—but expensive and complex—treatment regimes.

There has been a marked change in lifestyles in most of the countries as a result of urbanization, a sedentary lifestyle, and stress with an associated rise in the burden of noncommunicable diseases. A high prevalence of mental disorders has been observed in all the countries: seventeen million young people between the ages of four and sixteen years exhibit moderate or severe psychiatric disorder [5].

Environmental situation

Housing and basic domestic sanitation services are of paramount importance for health. The total housing deficit in Latin America and the Caribbean is estimated to be approximately fifty million dwellings [10]. Some nineteen million new dwellings are required and among the existing housing stock, twenty million, though habitable and reparable, are unhealthy; a further eleven million are beyond repair. The poorest housing conditions are found in rural and marginalized urban areas and almost all indigenous people live in unhealthy dwellings.

Seventy-three percent of the Region's population have domestic water supply. However, in rural areas only 41 percent have domestic drinking water, compared with 84 percent in urban areas. Among those who have domestic water supply, only 59 percent receive properly disinfected water.

Roughly 69 percent of the total population has access to wastewater disposal services, with 80 percent of the urban population and 40 percent or the rural population covered by them. This represents a very modest growth regarding this service since 1980 when the total coverage was 59 percent (78 percent in urban areas and 28 percent in rural areas) [11]. Approximately 70 percent of all the waste produced daily in the Region are collected, but only 30 percent are properly disposed. Various methods are used, but the most frequent is the sanitary landfill.

Pollution, especially from industrial activities, the burning of fuel, and transportation, is a growing problem that affects the entire population, although with varying degrees of exposure and risk. Poor areas are the most vulnerable because of their greater exposure to industrial and domestic waste. In urban areas, the burning of fossil fuels to generate energy for home heating, motor vehicles, and industrial processes constitute the main source of air pollution. Some 80,000 chemical substances are currently sold in the Region, and between 1000 and 2000 new substances are put on the market annually.

It is estimated that 100,000 out of the five million workplace accidents each year results in death. The total costs associated with these accidents, which exclude accidents in the informal sector, are between 10 and 15 percent of the regional GDP [5].

In summary, Latin American countries are facing significant changes in their demographic, social and epidemiological profiles. The epidemiological transition is well advanced and new problems such as injuries and AIDS are emerging as major causes of death and morbidity. These changes do not reach all social groups uniformly and inequalities persist among and within countries. Decreases in the proportion of many problems have not been sufficient to promote a drop in the absolute numbers of people affected by them.

Essential public health functions

There is much controversy about definition of public health and public health functions [12,13]. In 2000, the Pan American Health Organization

Box 7.1   PAHO's Essential Public Health Functions (EPHF) [14]

The Pan American Health Organization (PAHO) implemented the *Public Health in the Americas Initiative*, to improve the definition and measurement of the essential public health functions as the basis for improving public health practice and strengthening the steering role of the health authority at all levels of the State. Eleven Essential Public Health Functions (EPHF) were identified:

1. Health situation monitoring and analysis.
2. Public health surveillance, research and the control of risks and damages in public health.
3. Health promotion.
4. Social participation and empowerment of citizens for health.
5. Development of policy, planning and managerial capacity to support public health efforts and the steering role of the National Health Authority.
6. Public health regulation and enforcement.
7. Evaluation and promotion of equitable access to necessary health services.
8. Human resources development and training in public health.
9. Ensuring the quality of personal and population-based health services.
10. Research, development and implementation of innovative public health solutions.
11. Reducing the impact of emergencies and disasters on health.

identified eleven Essential Public Health Functions for which the State responsibility should be strengthened (Box 7.1). The situation in the Region concerning each of these functions is now summarized.

Health situation monitoring and analysis

Monitoring health status to identify health problems in the community health situation is developed to some extent by most countries in the region, although not necessarily routinely and in a proper manner.

There is wide disparity among countries in national politics regarding health information and informatics, as well as in technological infrastructure, investment and deployment of health information systems.

A survey conducted by PAHO in twenty-four Latin American and Caribbean countries showed that nearly all of them conduct systematic health data collections, making use of standards defined at the national level, and that most of these data are related to epidemiological surveillance and the services provided [5]. However, many problems were identified in the utilization of information systems, such as duplication and gaps in the information, dubious quality, and little use of information by health policy-makers and managers.

Public health surveillance, research and control of risks

This function relates to the capacity to conduct research and surveillance on epidemic outbreaks and patterns of communicable and noncommunicable diseases, accidents, and exposure to toxic substances or environmental agents harmful to health. In the 1990s, efforts were made to restructure national epidemiological surveillance systems in the Region; even so many of these systems are still inadequate. The PAHO regularly evaluates these surveillance systems [15].

Health promotion

Improvements in health care technology and health service delivery are not sufficient to meet the challenges presented by the health situation described. A broader range of activities across many sectors is required to promote individual and collective health, involving environmental protection, investments in water supply and sanitation services, housing conditions, waste collection and disposal and food protection. Health promotion policies also include health communication efforts and intersectoral strategies, such as the "healthy municipalities" and the "health-promoting schools" initiatives.

The Agenda 21 plan for environmental protection, recognized by world leaders after the United Nations Conference on Environment and Development held in Rio de Janeiro in 1992 (also called *Earth Summit*), represented a political commitment to the implementation of environmental and health protection policies [16]. However, most of the recent health reforms in Latin America and Caribbean have focused in health services financing and organization and have not succeeded in implementing a comprehensive approach to health promotion at the national level.

In the context of political democratization in the Region, societal participation and control are key elements in most health reform proposals, usually related to decentralization policies. Nevertheless, participation mechanisms are varied among countries and, in some cases their real implementation or effectiveness is not clear. Brazil is the only country that instituted a network of health councils at the three levels of government, municipal, state and federal, by a 1991 law, followed by a series of operational norms.

Development of policy, planning and managerial capacity

In order to achieve the goal of improving the health of the people, health authorities must appropriately formulate policies and develop adequate planning, regulatory and evaluative actions. In most Latin American and Caribbean countries the institutional capacity is insufficient to fulfill the required steering role.

In the first place, there are important issues concerning the workforce required to develop these actions. Appropriately trained public health personnel are lacking in many levels of the administration. Specific governmental health careers have not been established, and due to the current structural adjustment policies there is instability and high turnover among public health administrators. The effective practice of public health requires many civil servants. Unfortunately, the region faces a decrease in the incentives for working in governmental institutions and the labor conditions in the field are deteriorating.

Secondly, most of the health reform initiatives occurring in the region have a strong component of decentralization. Local health authorities and managers have to be trained to respond to the new functions. A greater number of trained public health staff is needed in newly established health administrative structures.

Third, increased participation of the private sector in the delivery of health services requires the strengthening of the regulatory capabilities of public health administrators, since inappropriate action can lead to an increase in health inequalities. While most industrialized countries exercise strict control over private practice in health sector, in Latin American and Caribbean countries these regulations are underdeveloped.

Public health regulation and enforcement

Environment protection laws and regulations were passed and enforced in many countries during the 1990s. Many specific agencies, commissions and even courts, were created for this purpose. Many countries launched anti-tobacco initiatives including advertising restrictions. Norms and regulations for protection against some toxic agents such as oil and asbestos have been presented.

New roles for the private sector in health care delivery led to the production of a new set of laws and norms related to their functioning, mainly devoted to the protection of consumers' rights. A few countries instituted regulatory agencies to coordinate this new governmental role.

Almost all countries in the Region adopted new drug regulations, although the scope and strength of the regulatory capacities vary between countries. Some countries are putting forward policies to promote the use of pharmaceutical generics, including the revision of intellectual property agreements for essential drugs, as with AIDS drugs in Brazil. Many legislative initiatives are now in place to protect special population groups, for example, children, adolescents, HIV positive people, handicapped and old-age people. Health professions and occupations are mainly regulated by professional bodies although formal laws and norms are increasingly being produced in the region.

Evaluation and promotion of equitable access to necessary health services

Inequities in access to health services are a common feature in Latin American and Caribbean countries. Although health systems in many countries represent an important commitment of financial, organizational, physical and human resources, they are still insufficient for the vast and diverse needs of the Region's population. Scarcity of resources related to economic adjustment processes and recent reforms, such as the increasing participation of the private sector in the area, pose new equity challenges to health authorities.

Besides financial constraints and broader economic and social inequalities that affect health conditions and policies, accurate information on access to health services is rare; it is thus difficult for the health authorities to implement adequate strategies to increase necessary health services delivery and reduce the inequalities in access. Existing data suggest that there are significant inequities in access among regions in the same country, among urban and rural populations, and among different social classes. These inequalities can be observed in every level of service complexity. In many countries the coverage and quality of prenatal care varies greatly according to woman's social and educational status, despite efforts by health authorities to improve access to primary health care. Proper diagnostic facilities, such as imaging services, are scarce or inadequately distributed in most of the Region's countries, sometimes reducing the opportunity for effective early intervention. The situation is even worse regarding more complex services which tend to be concentrated in the largest cities.

Improvements in access to health care in the Region depend on many factors. Some countries have made efforts to adopt innovative health care models, such as family doctors; others have adopted policies which aim at augmenting coverage in specific population groups or diseases. However, considering that the great majority of the Region's population is poor, targeting alone will not improve equity in access to health services because of the overlap of many health interventions. Implementation is required of health policies that guarantee universal access to all system levels and specific strategies directed to the more vulnerable groups.

Human resources development and training

Human resources development is one of the central elements in national health policies and health sector reforms. Recently, this area has experienced many changes most of which derive from broad economic and political determinants, such as globalization and State reform processes. Recent data suggest that between 1993 and 1996 there was a slowing in the growth, or even a decrease, in the percentage of health workers in relation to the total working population, revealing the impact of the adjustment process on the health sector.

The availability of health professionals varies among and within countries. The concentration of health professionals in large cities and in some specialties is a common problem to most of the countries. Unresolved issues in human resources development in the Region include: the limited capacity of authorities to plan and act upon human resources needs, and to improve health personnel distribution and performance; reduced budgets in public institutions resulting in a decrease in numbers of public positions for health workers and a drop in their remuneration; and the scarcity of professionals with credentials required by new health care management models.

Although public institutions remain the major health personnel employers in the Region, an increasing number of health personnel are combining their public functions with private practice. Recent state and health reform trends have led to significant changes in the health sector's labor market. Many countries have promoted reforms that deregulate, or increase the flexibility in labor relations, including the health sector. Changes observed in the sector include: a reduced number of permanent positions in public health institutions; changes in remuneration, such as public wages contraction, and introduction of incentives for productivity; growth of temporary contracts and third-parties hiring; and creation of new types of private associations, such as cooperatives and professional groups that sell services to health establishments.

Other relevant issues in health personal development are the education and training of the health workforce. Educational institutions, particularly universities, are usually remote from the needs of public health systems. For example, although is an increasing demand in many countries for personnel capable of performing functions at the primary care level, universities tend to encourage specialization. Continuing education of health personnel is either insufficient or inappropriate. An ongoing survey by PAHO [17] identified 110 training programs in Latin American. Only four countries presented more than ten programs: Argentina (fifteen), Brasil (twenty-four), Ecuador (twelve), and Mexico (twenty-three).

Ensuring the quality of personal and population-based health services

Most countries have licensing norms and regulations for health professionals, facilities, and drugs and equipments and devices. However, almost none have regular evaluative or quality improvement initiatives in place. Argentina, Colombia, Brazil and Mexico are implementing systems of health care evaluation for accreditation purposes, but these are mostly directed to hospitals. Some countries are adopting technical protocols or clinical guidelines to diminish the variation of practice among care providers and assist in improving the quality and safety of the care delivered.

Research, development and implementation of innovative public health solutions

It is estimated that Latin America and Caribbean account for only around 2 percent of the worldwide funding and scientific output in the health field. This health scientific output is highly concentrated in a few countries. Between 1973 and 1992, six countries—Argentina, Brazil, Chile, Cuba, Mexico and Venezuela—accounted for nearly 90 percent of all the Region's published articles, and among those more than 60 percent of the articles originated in Brazil and Argentina (33 and 28 percent, respectively). The data suggest that health research and scientific output in the Region is still extremely limited in quantitative terms, concentrated in few countries, and mostly researcher driven as opposed to targeted prioritized research [18].

Reducing the impact of emergencies and disasters on health

The population of Latin American and the Caribbean countries is often exposed to natural and human-made risks: seismic and volcanic activity in the Andean countries, Central America and Mexico; hurricanes in the Caribbean region; floods and landslides in most countries; and accidents caused by different types of hazardous materials (contaminations, explosions or transportation accidents). Many of these events have a greater affect on the poorest population groups.

International cooperation both in disaster preparedness and in relief operations have played an important role in establishing general recommendations and guidelines, disseminating information, and financing technical support to many countries. At the national level, some countries have instituted changes in their legal framework or official agencies, increased training activities, developed plans for preparing and repairing infrastructure systems, invested in structural and functional safety of health facilities, and made increased efforts in organizing humanitarian response. In some countries, however, poor living conditions in urban and rural areas still increase the risks of exposure to different types of disasters and the probability of serious damage as a consequence. Recent chemical and bioterrorism threats have required countries to review and improve their systems of preparedness, including systems of surveillance and laboratory capacity.

Public health challenges

The Summit of America's leaders in Quebec in April 2001 established guidelines for actions in the health sector and reaffirmed the "commitment to an equity-oriented health sector reform process, emphasizing their concerns for essential public health functions, quality of care, equal access to health services and health coverage especially in the fields of disease prevention and health promotion, and improving the use of resources and administration of health services" [19].

Market forces by themselves will not drive the appropriate response to cover the old or the emerging agenda of health problems in Latin America and Caribbean. Governments will have to play a central role in articulating economic and social policies oriented to re-engage a new era of development and to reduce social and regional inequalities. Multilateral agencies have a greater role to play in stimulating the cooperation among countries and in finding ways to deal with the debt burden, without imposing an extra burden upon socially and economically disadvantaged populations.

Sound national social policies for the protection of the poor and disadvantaged should be developed and implemented in an integrated way. Social protection networks involving governmental and nongovernmental institutions and groups must be built and expanded to support people in need. National social and health goals must underpin all economic policies and adjustment policies should not compromise progress in social security and welfare.

Health sector planning should be based on a sound epidemiological basis and priorities set according to the needs of the population. Effectiveness of proposed actions should always be taken into account when designing strategies for coping with the complexities of current health problems. Current undisclosed priorities must be uncovered, and priorities must be revised in order to assure that the targeted groups are the ones in most need and that resources are appropriately employed.

Decentralization of activities continues to be a major administrative goal in the region. However, adequate coordination and regional and national objectives must guide the process. Increased accountability to the public, associated with community participation and social control, is crucial to the achievement of the best results of public health initiatives. Information systems that continuously feed policymakers and health professionals must be developed and improved. Engagement of health personnel is crucial, in order to promote the required changes.

These objectives will necessitate a new wave of health reform initiatives that will require the leadership of health authorities at all political levels as well as mobilization of the public health community, health professionals and the public at large. The success or failure of the process must, as always, be measurable in terms of reduction of inequalities in health determinants, in access to health services, and in a sustained reduction of the burden of disease and suffering.

References

[1] Economic Commission for Latin America and the Caribbean. Changing macroeconomic challenges. *ECLAC Notes* 2001;15: 7–8.

[2] Economic Commission for Latin America and the Caribbean. A decade of light and shadow. *ECLAC Notes* 2001;15: 1–3.

[3] Ocampo JM. The pending agenda. *ECLAC Notes* 2001;**15**: 2.

[4] Economic Commission for Latin America and the Caribbean. Social panorama of Latin America 2000–2001. Santiago: ECLAC, 2001.

[5] Pan American Health Organization. Health in the Americas 1998 Edition. Washington: PAHO, 1998.

[6] Pan American Health Organization. Strategic and programmatic orientations for the Pan American Sanitary Bureau, 1999–2002. CE 122/8 (Eng.). 1998. Washington, PAHO. 112nd Session of the Executive Committee.

[7] Castillo-Salgado C, Mujica O, Loyola E. A Subregional Assessment of Demographic and Health Trends in the Americas: 1980–1998. *Metropolitan Life Insurance Company Statistical Bulletin* 1999; **80**(2).

[8] Pan American Health Organization. Health Analysis: Risk of dying and income inequalities. *PAHO Epidemiological Bulletin* 2002; **20**: 7–10.

[9] World Health Organization. *Injury. A Leading Cause of the Global Burden of Disease.* Geneva: WHO, 1999.

[10] Franco R. Los paradigmas de la política social en América Latina. *Revista de la CEPAL* 1996; **58**: 9–22.

[11] Pan American Health Organization. *Mid-Decade Evaluation of Water Supply and Sanitation in Latin America and the Caribbean.* 1997. Washington, PAHO.

[12] Institute of Medicine. *The Future of Public Health.* Washington: National Academy Press, 1988.

[13] Pan American Health Organization. *The Crisis of Public Health: Reflections for the Debate.* Washington: PAHO, 1992.

[14] Pan American Health Organization. Essential Public Health Functions. CD42/15 (Eng.). 2000. Washington, PAHO. 42nd Directing Council. 52nd Session of the Regional Committee.

[15] Pan American Health Organization. Public Health surveillance in the Americas: national epidemiological surveillance and statistical information systems. PAHO. 2000. http://www.paho.org/English/SHA/shavsp.htm (1-12-2002).

[16] United Nations. Earth Summit. Agenda 21: The United Nations programme of action from Rio. New York: United Nations, 1992.

[17] Godue C. Public health training in Latin America. Pan American Health Organization. 2002. Personal Communication.

[18] Brasil. Ministerio da Ciencia e Tecnologia. Ciencia, tecnologia e inovação: desafio para a sociedade brasileira. Brasilia: Ministerio da Ciencia e Tecnologia, 2001.

[19] Pan American Health Organization. Report on the third Summit of the Americas. CD 43/16 (Eng.). 2001. Washington, PAHO. 43rd Directing Council. 53rd Session of the Regional Committee.

Chapter 8

Public health in Africa

David Sanders, Delanyo Dovlo, Wilma
Meeus and Uta Lehmann

Introduction

This chapter addresses public health issues relevant to sub-Saharan Africa
(SSA). SSA comprises forty-eight countries; it excludes Egypt, Libya,
Tunisia, Algeria and Morocco.

Health status and services in SSA

Notwithstanding improvements in health status that have occurred in SSA
over the last fifty years, the current situation on the continent is of great
concern, despite the paucity and unreliability of health data, as shown in
the annexed table (Annex 1).

In 1999, seven of the forty-eight SSA countries had a lower life expectancy
(LE) than in 1970, while eight countries have seen an increase in infant
mortality rate (IMR) between 1981 and 1999. Life expectancy in seventeen
of forty-eight countries declined between 1981 and 1999, probably through
a combination of average per capita incomes of less than US$1 per day,
the impact of the HIV epidemic, declines in health service provision, and
conflict.

1. Fourteen of the seventeen countries where LE decreased have a high
   prevalence of HIV, affecting in particular the 15–45 age range. The number of HIV infected people in SSA is estimated at twenty-eight million,
   approximately 70 percent of the total of HIV infected people globally [1].

2. Thirteen of forty-eight SSA countries have been or are still involved in
   conflict, while neighboring countries are affected by the conflicts because
   of population movements across international borders. The breakdown

of the delivery of most social services, including health care, is a frequent accompaniment of conflict.

3. Twenty-eight of forty-eight countries had an average per capita income of less than $1 per day in 1999, compared to nineteen of thirty-six countries in 1981. The GDP data are aggregates that do not show the increasing gap between the rich and the poor within countries.

Disaggregation of infant, under-five mortality and life expectancy data reveals that the gap in mortality rates between rich and poor countries has widened significantly: the relative probability of dying for under-5-year-olds in developing countries compared to western and eastern European countries increased from a ratio of 3.4 in 1950 to 8.8 in 1990 [2]. Similarly, improvements in health status have been slower in SSA as shown in Table 8.1.

The past two decades have witnessed an alarming resurgence and spread of "old" communicable diseases once thought to be well controlled, for example, cholera, tuberculosis, malaria, yellow fever and trypanosomiasis, while "new" epidemics, notably HIV/AIDS, threaten last century's health gains in many developing countries, but especially in SSA.

To aggravate matters, many developing countries are experiencing an "epidemiological transition", with cardiovascular diseases, cancers, diabetes, other chronic conditions and trauma, replacing communicable diseases in some social groups, but in others, co-existing with them. This in reality constitutes an epidemiological polarization, with poorer sectors

Table 8.1 Decline in Infant Mortality Rate (IMR) and Under-five Mortality Rate (UMR) between 1960, 1981 and 1999

Indicator	IMR 1960	IMR 1981	Decline 1960–81	Percent decline 1960–81	IMR 1999	Decline 1981–99	Percent decline 1981–99
World	127	78	49	38.5	57	21	26.9
SSA	156	126	30	19.2	107	19	15.1
	UMR 1960	UMR 1981	Decline 1960–81	Percent decline 1960–81	UMR 1999	Decline 1981–99	Percent decline 1981–99
World	198	91	107	54.0	82	9	9.9
SSA	258	203	55	21.3	173	30	14.8

Source: UNICEF's State of the World's Children—1984 [3], 1994 [4], 2001 [5].

of the population experiencing high child mortality and morbidity as well as a high burden of noncommunicable disease [6]. In South Africa, for example, children from poor families still suffer mainly from infectious diseases, whereas increasing rates of hypertension, chronic lung diseases and diabetes affect the urban, and especially poorer, adult population [7].

Access to health services improved considerably during the period 1980–90, but has worsened since then as shown by Expanded Programme on Immunization (EPI) coverage data (Table 8. 2). The EPI coverage data for SSA in 1999 show declines in coverage of all routinely administered antigens. This occurred despite the intensive polio vaccination campaigns and the regular measles vaccination campaigns. In addition, nutrition is deteriorating, access to water is low (only 40 percent of rural SSA—constituting 60 percent of SSA—populations had access to adequate water supplies in 1999 [5]) as is access to good sanitation, particularly by rural populations. It is not surprising that the health situation is deteriorating in a number of countries.

Many countries have also been unable to significantly reallocate resources from tertiary and specialized services to basic health services or find increased resources to moderate the imbalance, despite warnings given as early as the mid-1960s [8]. In Ghana, for instance, only 42 percent of the health budget is allocated to district level health service delivery, while the central Ministry of Health's budget allocation amounts to 16 percent, tertiary facilities use almost 20 percent and regional level services use 23 percent of the national health budget [9]. Most SSA countries still spend less than an average US$10 per person on health care, an amount that is 20–40 percent below the frugal amount considered necessary to cover the basic package of health services recommended by the World Bank [10].

Education indicators show that 54 percent of women are still functionally illiterate in SSA in 1999, as compared to 31 percent globally. In SSA, 33 percent of girls were not enrolled in primary school in 1999 despite the many efforts made to make primary education accessible to all children [5].

In summary, gains in health status in SSA and access to health and related services have been slower than elsewhere in the world, even compared to other developing regions. Given the much weaker starting point of SSA countries, it is disturbingly apparent that some of the gains of the past twenty years are being reversed. These developments are partly explained by public health policy and governance trends. In the following sections we briefly outline how public health policies and services have evolved in SSA since the end of the colonial period and how they have been influenced by globalization.

Table 8.2 EPI coverage (percentage of fully vaccinated one year old children)

	BCG 1980	BCG 1990	Change 1980–90	BCG 1999	Change 1990–99
World	58	79	+21	81	+2
SSA	46	72	+26	65	−7
	DPT 3—1980	DPT 3—1990	Change 1980–90	DPT 3—1999	Change 1990–99
World	44	74	+30	75	+1
SSA	30	55	+25	50	−5
	Polio 3—1980	Polio 3—1990	Change 1980–90	Polio 3—1999	Change 1990–99
World	46	75	+29	76	+1
SSA	25	54	+29	50	−4
	Measles—1980	Measles—1990	Change 1980–90	Measles—1999	Change 1990–99
World	39	75	+36	72	−3
SSA	37	58	+21	51	−7

Source: UNICEF's State of the World's Children—1984 [3], 1994 [4], 2001 [5].

Trends in development of public health services

Changes in health policies and their context in SSA

The SSA economic and political history has been tied into the world economy for the past 500 years, starting with the slave trade in the sixteenth century. Colonization tightened and formalized these ties and European administrative systems dislodged, suppressed and reinvented indigenous systems and traditions. Newly independent African states took over a racialized, colonial state machinery, which had to be Africanized with an extremely weak human resource base. For instance, in Tanzania in 1962 only sixteen of 184 physicians, one of eighty-four civil engineers, and two of fifty-seven lawyers were Africans [11]. In a number of countries rebuilding and restructuring attempts ground to a halt with the 1970s oil crisis and the worldwide economic recession which followed. This recession was precipitated by the stringent financial policies adopted by the northern countries (particularly the United States and the United Kingdom) from the early 1980s, involving tight credit, high interest rates and reductions in government spending. The resulting economic slowdown was passed on to the developing countries through reduced demand for exports and cuts in foreign aid [12]. Together with deteriorating terms of trade, this led to a reversal in the flow of capital with developing countries becoming net exporters of capital and acquiring huge debts.

Health sector policies in post-colonial SSA

Newly independent African states, as a rule, inherited patchy and highly uneven health care systems which they sought to restructure in different ways. While most tried to build health systems that would better serve disadvantaged areas, the majority of government and international funding continued to go to curative, urban services [13]. There were exceptions, such as Tanzania, following the 1967 Arusha Declaration, and later Mozambique under the Frelimo government [14], both of which promoted a strategy emphasizing community-based health care. A significant post-colonial development was the expansion of rural health centers staffed by auxiliaries such as medical and health assistants which improved health service coverage. However, by the mid-1970s these early efforts to reshape health care delivery and governance were severely undermined by the economic recession which resulted in a dramatic shortage of resources to invest in health care, education and social services.

The era of primary health care

These setbacks contributed to a growing realization internationally that the provision of health care for all would need a fundamental and systemic rethinking of health care strategies [15]. This culminated in the 1978 Alma Ata Declaration on Primary Health Care (PHC) which stressed the need for community-based, affordable and accessible health care for all. The Declaration also placed health within its social, economic and political context, calling for an equitable distribution of resources. However, the following years saw a move to "selective Primary Health Care", [16] with a continued focus on vertical programmes and selected, technical interventions, eschewing comprehensive, multisectoral and integrated health care provision. This trend was nurtured by the prevailing conservative political ideology of the 1980s which de-emphasized the broader determinants of health such as income inequalities, the environment, community development, and emphasized health care technologies [17].

There were some significant successes in selective PHC, particularly in the 1980s. The most impressive achievements have been in child health care provision with the vigorous promotion of selected "Child Survival" technologies such as growth monitoring, oral rehydration therapy, breast-feeding and immunization. Of these, immunization improved most dramatically, with global coverage of one year old children increasing from 20 percent in 1980 to 80 percent by 1990 [18].

Selective PHC was reinforced by the World Bank's 1993 World Development Report, "Investing in Health", [19] which recognized the importance of health to development. Based on calculations of burden of disease, it specified the most cost-effective health interventions, and formulated a core package of health services to be provided at the different levels of care. The identification of core packages has become a rationing mechanism to control the cost of health services provided by the state. This reflected the Bank's wider economic and fiscal policies, encouraging the privatization of health care delivery and the cutting back of state services.

At the start of the twenty-first century an assessment of progress is sobering. Apart from falling vaccination coverage and rising IMRs, evaluations have raised questions about the sustainability of mass vaccination campaigns [20], the effectiveness of health facility-based growth monitoring [21] and the appropriateness of ORT when promoted as sachets or packets and without a corresponding emphasis on nutrition, water and sanitation [13]. For example, although Ethiopia has managed to increase polio vaccination coverage to approximately 80 percent in 2001 from less than 10 percent in 1992, largely as a result of vaccination campaigns, five suspected cases of polio have been reported recently in a remote area [22]. A systematic review has pointed out the lack of evidence for the effectiveness of directly observed therapy for TB (DOTS) in the absence of well functioning health services and community engagement [23]. Only when these core service activities are embedded in a more comprehensive approach (which includes paying attention to social equity, health systems and human capacity development), are real and sustainable improvements in the health status of populations seen [24 25].

The concept of district health systems (DHS) emerged in response to the fact that, almost a decade after Alma Ata, the activities of various programmes and institutions continued to be piecemeal and poorly co-ordinated. In 1986 the District Health System concept was officially adopted by the World Health Organization (WHO) Global Programme Committee [26]. Tanzania had started devolving responsibilities to district health teams in the early 1980s and only had to re-align some of the aspects of its implementation, while Zimbabwe had made great strides in implementing health districts by 1987. Other countries, such as South Africa, Burkina Faso and Malawi started DHS implementation in the mid-1990s.

The district was identified as "the natural meeting point for bottom-up planning and organization and top-down planning and support". [27] It is the place where community needs and national priorities could be reconciled and the most appropriate level for the organization and management of services to communities.

In many countries, however, devolution of management of health services was not accompanied by adequate resources and authority and in some cases did not involve decentralization to elected local governments. Where decentralization occurred, local government at times did not have control over the health sector, as happened in Ghana. In Uganda, however, health service management was devolved significantly to local government, but resulted in the health sector receiving less financial resources than the government would have allocated [28].

Globalization, health and health services in SSA

The increased mobility of capital and labour and cheaper cost of communication have accelerated pre-existing economic, political and social interdependence which characterizes the modern phase of globalization. The most important early interventions further integrated developing countries into the global economy, primarily through the imposition of stringent debt repayments and the liberalization of trade. Of particular importance have been Structural Adjustment Programmes (SAPs) promoted by the International Monetary Fund (IMF) and the World Bank. SAPs have also resulted in significant macro-economic policy changes and public sector restructuring and reduced social provisioning, with negative effects on education, health and social services for the poor. A recent review of available studies on structural adjustment and health for a WHO commission states: "The majority of studies in Africa, whether theoretical or empirical, are negative towards structural adjustment and its effects on health outcomes". [29]

More recently, other instruments of globalization have further undermined the ability of developing country governments to provide health care for their populations. For example, the development of agreements under the World Trade Organisation (WTO), notably the Agreement on Trade-Related Intellectual Property Rights (TRIPS) and its interpretation by powerful corporate interests and governments, have threatened to circumscribe countries' health policy options. The best known case relates to the recent legal battle around the attempt by South Africa to secure pharmaceuticals, especially for HIV/AIDS, at a reduced cost. In 1997 Nelson Mandela signed into legislation a law aimed at lowering drug prices through "parallel importing"—that is importing drugs from countries where they are sold at lower prices—and "compulsory licensing", which would allow local companies to manufacture certain drugs, in exchange for royalties. Both provisions are legal under the TRIPS agreement as all sides agreed that HIV/AIDS is an emergency. This was confirmed during the WTO meeting in Doha in 2001. The US administration did not bring its case to the WTO but instead, acting in concert with the multinational pharmaceutical corporations, brought a number of pressures (e.g., threats of trade sanctions and legal action) to bear on the South African Government to rescind the legislation. This followed similar successful threats against Thailand and Bangladesh [30]. However, an uncompromising South African Government, together with a vigorous campaign mounted by local and international AIDS activists and progressive health NGOs, forced a climb-down by both the US government and the multinational pharmaceutical companies [31].

Notwithstanding this important victory, the provisions of the WTO, particularly TRIPS and the General Agreement on Trade in Services hold many threats for the health of developing countries' economies and their citizens [32]. This was succinctly noted in a recent speech by President Museveni of Uganda: "It (globalization) is the same old order with new means of control, new means of oppression, new means of marginalization". [33]

Reforming health sector governance

The rapidly changing economic policy environment has been accompanied by an equally unstable organizational and governance environment. The development of district health systems was followed in the early 1990s by the concept of health sector reform (HSR) which introduced a comprehensive framework for government's health sector policy development, strategies, structures and systems under conditions of increasing fiscal austerity. The HSR package includes, in most cases, the following component areas [15, 34]:

- improvement of performance of the civil service;
- decentralization of management responsibility and/or provision of health care to local level;
- improvement of national ministry of health's functioning;
- broadening health financing options—e.g., user fees, insurance schemes; introduction of managed competition between providers of clinical and support services'
- working with the private sector through contracting, regulating and franchising different service providers.

A number of SSA countries are currently undergoing reforms (Ghana, Ethiopia, Tanzania, Zambia, Uganda, Malawi). In Ghana e.g., the key principles enunciated in the Medium Term Health Strategy revolve around improving equity of access to health services, improving the efficiency with which resources for health are allocated and utilized, improving the effectiveness and quality of interventions, and incorporating and co-ordinating all stakeholders, consumers and service providers in the decisions for prioritizing services and utilizing resources. These principles partly respond to significant pressure to shift aspects of service delivery to NGOs and other private sector providers. However, their implementation has been piecemeal and of limited success in promoting greater health equity [35].

Human resources for health: A key challenge

The deteriorating economic environment and unstable organizational context have also impacted very negatively on the health workforce, leading in turn to deterioration in the quality of health care. Key problems in SSA include:

(1) inherited professional cadres and health care structures fashioned for Western health systems, which were inappropriate for African health needs;

(2) inability to build adequate capacity within Ministries of Health and health services to manage new strategies and systems in a constantly changing policy environment;

(3) increasing workloads of health workers caused by fiscal constraints (vacant posts being frozen), the restructuring of services and the impact of the HIV/AIDS epidemic;

(4) low productivity and motivation of health workers due to the above factors, leading to poor service delivery and high rates of absenteeism and migration out of the system.

Inappropriate professional cadres and structures

Africa suffers from very low health worker/population ratios [36]. Furthermore, the orientation of many health professionals remains more appropriate to the service needs of industrialized countries and better-off populations. As in industrialized countries, public health remains a marginal area of professional health activity: the numbers of health personnel with any significant public health training are tiny.

In many SSA countries, tertiary health facilities (teaching and specialist hospitals) have continued to retain high proportions of the health budget. These general trends in resource allocation have contributed to a mal-distribution of staff, who prefer to work in well-resourced tertiary care facilities and in urban areas. Eventually, as these facilities have also deteriorated, they have joined the brain drain into the private sector or to other countries [37].

To achieve better coverage of their populations, countries such as Ghana, Tanzania and Malawi introduced country-specific cadres such as medical assistants and clinical officers to whom were delegated some of the tasks carried out by doctors. These cadres were better retained in rural areas and in primary health care services. Other countries such as Ethiopia developed cadres such as field surgeons to deal with the consequences of war and they have been integrated into the health system. Despite the impact these cadres have made in improving the coverage of services in underserved areas, their training and development have often not received adequate investment.

Inability to develop appropriate capacity

Capacity problems have been experienced at various levels. Few health workers have had training in areas of public health such as health systems management at the district level (e.g., planning, budgeting, financial and human resource management, monitoring and evaluation). Capacity problems have, for example, been blamed for slow implementation of reforms in Ethiopia [38] necessitating use of external technical assistance. The WHO supported "Strengthening District Health Systems" initiative in Ghana and Zambia is one effort made to bridge the gap between planning and implementation in districts. However, such initiatives often revealed the lack of supervisory support needed to sustain implementation.

Attempts have also been made to restructure Ministries of Health in order to prepare them to better support the operational levels. Despite restructuring efforts, human resource development and retention have suffered in many countries, blunting the implementation or achievement of health goals. Retention and motivation have become major issues for service delivery in Africa and it is recognised that most reform initiatives have tackled human resources issues mainly from the viewpoint of reducing costs by cutting staffing levels. An independent review of the Zambian Health Reforms [39] noted that human resources issues were not treated as a major priority. The resulting workload increase and the perceived shift of resources and patients to the private sector have exacerbated the frustrations of staff.

The brain drain of health professionals

The haemorrhage of health professionals from African countries is easily the single most serious human resource problem facing health ministries today. This drain occurs from developing countries to the developed world but also to the relatively better-off developing countries. For example, South Africa, despite its own emigration problems, is the recipient of large numbers of doctors from other African countries. Some 20 percent of doctors (approximately 6000) on the South African Medical Register in 1999 were expatriates [40]. The brain drain has hit some countries very severely [41–43].

The recipient countries of the "brain drain" are few. Agreements to manage the process and the numbers as well as the involvement of the "exporting" countries in the recruitment and selection process could ameliorate the situation and ensure some remittance of earnings. For example, in 1996 and 1998 Ghana's Ministry of Health entered into agreements with the Ministry of Health in Jamaica and with some recruitment agencies in the United Kingdom, aimed mainly at restricting numbers recruited so as to avoid collapse of services and to ensure return after an agreed period [40].

Almost all countries in SSA have expatriate health workers. The poorer countries often have NGO service providers while the richer recruit health workers from neighbouring countries. The commonest formal inter-government agreement is that with the government of Cuba for doctors and other medical personnel. The Cuban Medical Brigades are found in a number of countries including Ghana, South Africa and Namibia [40].

HIV/AIDS and human resources in Africa

The HIV/AIDS epidemic sweeping the continent is already affecting the health workforce significantly. These effects include reduction in trained personnel through death, as indicated by the higher than usual death rates among some health personnel in Malawi [37]. Other effects expressed anecdotally include "burn-out" and high rates of early leavers from the services, absenteeism to attend funerals and illness, all of which are aggravated by the existing service conditions in many countries.

In summary, economic decline, structural adjustment and health sector reform in combination with the consequences of the HIV epidemic and continued conflict in a number of countries, have adversely affected the capacity of SSA health systems to provide comprehensive health services to their populations. Health human resource requirements are unmet, both in terms of coverage and relevant skills. Moreover, many SSA countries continue to be embroiled in conflicts resulting in complex emergencies and affecting livelihoods and increasing demand for health care, while health service delivery is disrupted.

Perspectives for the future

The Global Fund to Fight AIDS, Tuberculosis and Malaria: An opportunity and a threat for SSA

In recognition of the growing global health divide between North and South and the crisis imposed by HIV/AIDS and the resurgence of TB and malaria in the South, the UN Secretary General announced in 2001 the establishment of a Global Fund. While this initiative is welcome there is a need for the mixed experience outlined above of health policy implementation of the past twenty years to inform the utilisation of these new resources. As a recent editorial stated: "The dominant fear ... was that this new public–private partnership fund would (yet again) be donor led. As a result undue emphasis would be put on supplying drugs rather than building up capacity to implement and sustain effective treatment and preventive programmes". [44]

This view is reinforced by a recent review of health systems in Africa, which concludes that: "Programmes to tackle these important diseases will not be sustainable in the long-run unless effective health services are in place. International aid should therefore support system development and improve the delivery of health services". [10] These concerns are reminiscent of the critical response from within the Health for All movement to selective PHC, and are supported by worrying evidence concerning the sustainability of the selected child survival interventions which received external resources and for which great progress was achieved in the 1980s. A sustainable response to the considerable health challenges of SSA must include a development strategy which addresses the strengthening of seriously weakened health systems.

Sector Wide Approaches as a mechanism to reduce donor imposition

Sector Wide Approaches (SWAps) are a response to the limitations of development assistance and the practical expression of partnerships between governments and donors. Their aim is twofold. First, to facilitate the efficiency of resource generation, allocation and utilisation. Second, to improve the effectiveness of service delivery by encouraging government leadership of policy formulation and priority setting for the sector, recognition and involvement of all stakeholders in the sector (especially development partners) in policy development, implementation and monitoring, and better co-ordination of all resources of the sector. SWAps particularly aim to give governments a stronger role in co-ordinating external support and allowing a sustained partnership between government and all its partners [45].

A number of countries (Ethiopia, Ghana and Mali) have made progress in the development of comprehensive health plans that include clear targets for the medium term. Similar processes are nearly finalized in Burkina Faso and Mozambique [46]. The ability of SWAps to better respond to national priorities will probably depend on the capacity and ability of countries to retain control of the process and to adequately implement plans and competently manage the allocated funds [47].

A strategy for health systems development [15]

Countries which have achieved the greatest and most durable improvements in health tend to be those with a commitment to equitable and broad-based development, and to health systems that are comprehensive and engage related sectors. Good empirical evidence for this comes from a number of countries, including some poor developing countries, for example, the "Good Health at Low Cost" models of Sri Lanka, China, Costa Rica and Kerala State in India. These countries demonstrate that investment in the social sectors, and particularly in women's education, health and welfare, can have a significant positive impact on the health and social indicators of the whole population [24].

The World Bank recently introduced Poverty Reduction Strategy Papers (PRSPs) as the basis for financing comprehensive poverty reduction strategies in Highly Indebted Poor Countries. Uganda is the first of twenty-six countries that have signed PRSP agreements and is to receive a US$ 150 million loan to support the implementation of the poverty reduction strategy with the goal of improving the delivery of basic services to the population.

PRSP's are aimed at strengthening country ownership of poverty reduction strategies, broadening representation of civil society in the design of strategies, and improving co-ordination among development partners so as to focus the resources of the international community on achieving results in reducing poverty. However, as Verheul and Rowson suggest "Systems to collect data to monitor poverty reduction are crude, government policies fragmented, and public servants demoralized. Countries such as Rwanda do not have their own technical capacity to collect and analyse data, while the scant national budgets of Benin or Mali offer little real prospect of reform". [48]

Of continuing and pressing relevance to the challenge of health development in SSA is the need for integrated and sustainable comprehensive health systems [49]. Comprehensive health systems comprise curative and rehabilitative components to address the effects of health problems, a preventive component to address the immediate and underlying causative factors which operate at the level of the individual, and a promotive component which addresses the more basic (intersectoral) causes which operate at the level of society.

The principles of comprehensive programme development apply to all health problems, including HIV, TB and malaria. Much experience has been gained internationally in the development of comprehensive and integrated programmes to combat under-nutrition; these experiences can provide useful lessons for other programmes [50].

After the priority health problems in a district or local area have been identified, the first step in programme development is a situation analysis. This should identify the prevalence and distribution of the problem, its causes, and potential resources, including community capacities and strengths, which can be mobilized and actions which can be undertaken to address the problem. The more effective programmes have taken this approach, involving health workers, workers from other sectors and the community in the three phases of programme development: assessment of the nature and extent of the problem, analysis of its multilevel causation and action to address the linked causes.

The specific combination of actions making up a comprehensive programme will vary from situation to situation. The inclusion of a set of health service activities should constitute the core of a comprehensive control strategy e.g., DOTS for TB, early treatment of STDs, promotion of condom usage and prevention of mother to child transmission for HIV, and effective prophylaxis and treatment and impregnated bed nets for malaria. For these activities to be sustained they need to be embedded within functioning health systems and complemented by relevant promotive policies and activities in health related sectors (e.g., improved housing and nutrition for TB, life skills education for HIV prevention, and environmental improvements for malaria).

The development of comprehensive and integrated health systems requires transformation of both management and practice. A broadening and deepening of public health competencies is urgently required [51]. A key primary step is capacity development through training and guided health systems research which must be practice-based and problem-oriented, and draw upon and simultaneously re-orientate educational institutions and professional bodies. The successful development of decentralised health systems will require targeted investment in infrastructure, personnel and management and information systems. For instance in South Africa, the University of the Western Cape developed a model Health Information System Programme (HISP) that was adopted by the Department of Health for implementation throughout the country after it proved successful in the districts of one province. The Ministries of Health of Mozambique and Ghana have also adopted the HISP.

The WHO Regional Office for Africa has indicated the importance of setting Human Resource (HR) Development as a priority and in 1998 developed the Regional Strategy for development of Human Resources for health [52]. Progress in implementing this strategy has included formation of a Multi-Disciplinary Advisory Group on Human Resources for Health and a plan of action [53]; countries have been assisted to develop HR Plans and Policies and a number of tools, advocacy packs and guidelines are under development.

The shift in focus from selective disease specific interventions to a more comprehensive health systems approach implies a shift in policy emphasis, time horizons and scale and duration of investment. To secure sustained investment in the health and social sectors and the equity essential for a healthy society, evidence suggests that a strong, organised demand for government responsiveness and accountability to social needs is crucial [54]. Tacit recognition of this important dynamic informed the Alma Ata call for strong community participation. To achieve and sustain the political will to meet all people's basic needs, and to regulate the activities of the private sector, a process of participatory democracy—or at least a well-informed movement of civil society—is essential. "Strong" community participation is important not only in securing greater government responsiveness to social needs but also in providing an active, conscious and organised population so critical to the design, implementation and sustainability of comprehensive health systems.

The Global Fund to Fight AIDS, Tuberculosis and Malaria presents an opportunity to African countries to mount a response to their health crises. However, unless these resources contribute to the development of infrastructure, human capacity and management processes, the response is likely to have only a short-term impact on Africa's pressing health problems.

Annex 1

Changes in:

+ life expectancy at birth (LE) between 1970, 1981 and 1999;
+ Infant Mortality Rate (IMR) between 1960, 1981 and 1999;
+ per capita GDP (in US$) between 1981, 1992 and 1999;
+ countries with average per capita income of less than US$ 1/ per day (1999).

Country	Average per capita income <$1/day, 1999	LE			IMR			GDP per capita (US$)		
		70	81	99	60	81	99	81	92	99
Angola	Y	37	42	48	210	150	_172_	490	610	220
Benin		43	50	54	210	150	99	320	380	380
Botswana		**52**	**57**	**45**	**120**	**80**	**46**	**1010**	**2530**	**3240**
Burkina Faso	Y	39	44	45	250	210	106	240	290	240
Burundi	**Y**	**44**	**45**	**43**	**150**	**120**	**106**	**230**	**210**	**120**
Cameroon		44	50	54	160	110	95	880	850	580
Cape Verde		57	68 (1992)	70	110	44 (1992)	_54_	—	750	1330
CAR	Y	42	43	45	200	150	113	320	390	290
Chad	Y	38	43	48	200	150	118	110	210	200
Comoros	Y	48	56 (1992)	60	165	90 (1992)	64	—	500	350
Congo		**46**	**60**	**49**	**140**	**130**	**81**	**1110**	**1120**	**670**
Cote d'Ivoire		44	47	47	170	120	102	1200	690	710
DRC	Y	45	50	52	150	110	_128_	210	230	110
Djibouti		40	49 (1992)	51	186	113 (1992)	104	—	1210	790
Equat Guinea		40	48 (1992)	51	188	118 (1992)	105	—	330	1170
Eritrea	Y	43	47 (1992)	51	170	—	66	—	120	200
Ethiopia	**Y**	**40**	**46**	**44**	**180**	**150**	**118**	**140**	**120**	**100**

Country	Average per capita income <$1/day, 1999	LE	LE	LE	IMR	IMR	IMR	GDP per capita (US$)	GDP per capita (US$)	GDP per capita (US$)
Gabon		**44**	**53 (1992)**	**52**	**171**	**95 (1992)**	**85**	**—**	**3780**	**3350**
Gambia	Y	36	45 (1992)	48	207	133 (1992)	61	—	360	340
Ghana		49	54	61	140	100	63	400	400	390
Guinea		37	43	47	210	160	115	300	460	510
Guinea Biss.	Y	36	43 (1992)	45	190	150	128	—	180	160
Kenya	**Y**	**50**	**56**	**51**	**140**	**80**	**76**	**420**	**340**	**360**
Lesotho		48	52	54	140	110	93	540	580	550
Liberia	**Y**	**46**	**54**	**50**	**190**	**150**	**157**	**330**	**210**	**250**
Madagascar	Y	45	48	58	210	70	95	330	210	250
Malawi	**Y**	**40**	**44**	**40**	**210**	**170**	**132**	**200**	**230**	**190**
Mali	Y	42	45	54	200	150	143	190	280	240
Mauritania		43	44	54	190	140	120	460	510	380
Mauritius		62	65	72	70	34	19	1270	2410	3590
Mozambique	**Y**	**42**	**49**	**42**	**160**	**110**	**127**	**230**	**80**	**230**
Namibia		**47**	**58 (1992)**	**48**	**129**	**62 (1992)**	**56**	**—**	**1460**	**1890**
Niger	Y	38	45	49	190	140	162	330	300	190
Nigeria	Y	43	49	50	180	130	112	870	340	310
Rwanda	**Y**	**44**	**46**	**41**	**150**	**140**	**110**	**250**	**270**	**250**

Table *continued*

Country	Average per capita income <$1/day, 1999	LE		IMR			GDP per capita (US$)		
S Tome & Principe	Y	—	68 (1992)	—	65 (1992)	59	—	400	270
Senegal		41	44	180	140	68	430	720	510
Seychelles		—	71 (1992)	—	16 (1992)	13	—	5110	6540
Sierra Leone	Y	**34**	**47**	**230**	**200**	**182**	**320**	**210**	**130**
Somalia	Y	40	39	180	150	125	280	150	120
South Africa		**53**	**63**	**140**	**90**	**54**	**2770**	**2560**	**3160**
Sudan	Y	43	47	170	120	67	380	420	330
Swaziland		46	58 (1992)	157	74 (1992)	62	—	1050	1360
Tanzania	Y	**45**	**52**	**150**	**100**	**90**	**280**	**100**	**240**
Togo	Y	44	48	180	110	80	380	410	320
Uganda	Y	**46**	**48**	**140**	**100**	**83**	**220**	**170**	**320**
Zambia	Y	**46**	**51**	**150**	**100**	<u>**112**</u>	**600**	**420**	**320**
Zimbabwe		**50**	**55**	**120**	**70**	**60**	**870**	**650**	**520**

Bold: Countries with decrease in LE; **<u>Bold & underlined</u>**: countries with increase in IMR.

Source: UNICEF's State of the World's Children—1984 [3], 1994 [4] 2001 [5].

References

[1] Collins J, Rau B. AIDS in the Context of Development. Programme on Social Policy and Development, Paper number 4. Geneva: UNRISD, 2000.

[2] Legge DM. Investing in the shaping of world health policy. Paper presented at AIDAB, NCEPH and PHA Workshop to discuss Investing in Health, 31 August 1993. Canberra: 1993.

[3] UNICEF. *State of the World's Children. 1984.* Oxford: Oxford University Press, 1983.

[4] UNICEF. *State of the World's Children.* 1994. Oxford: Oxford University Press, 1993.

[5] UNICEF. *State of the World's Children.* Oxford: Oxford University Press, 2000.

[6] Frenk J, Bobadilla JL, Sepulveda J, Lopez Cervantes M. Health Transition in Middle-income Countries: New Challenges for Health Care. *Health Pol Planning* 1989; **4**: 29–39.

[7] South African Demographic and Health Survey. Preliminary report. Medical Research Council, Department of Health, MACRO International Inc., 1998.

[8] King M (ed.) *Medical Care in Developing Countries. A Symposium from Makerere.* Oxford: Oxford University Press, 1966.

[9] Addai E, Gaere L. Capacity-building and systems development for Sector-Wide Approaches (SWAps): the experience of the Ghana health sector. Ghana: MOH & DFID, 2001 (unpublished).

[10] Simms C, Rowson M, Peattie S. The Bitterest Pill of All. The collapse of Africa's health systems. London: Medact/Save the Children Briefing report, 2001.

[11] Iliffe J. *A Modern History of Tanganyika.* Cambridge: Cambridge University Press, 1979.

[12] Raghavan C. "What is globalisation?" *Third World Resurgence* 1996; **74**: 11–14.

[13] Werner D, Sanders D. *Questioning the Solution: The Politics of Primary Health Care and Child Survival.* Palo Alto, USA: Healthwrights, 1997.

[14] Zwi A, Mills A. Health policy in Less developed Countries. *J Int Development* 1995; **7**: 302–3.

[15] Sanders D. PHC 21—Everybody's business. Main background paper for the meeting: PHC 21—Everybody's business, An international meeting to celebrate 20 years after Alma Ata, Almaty, Kazakhstan, 27–28 November 1998. Geneva: WHO Report WHO/EIP/OSD/00.7, 1998.

[16] Rifkin SB, Walt G. Why health improves: defining the issues concerning "comprehensive primary health care" and "selective primary health care". *Soc Sci Med* 1986; **23**: 559–66.

[17] Chopra M, Sanders D, McCoy D, Cloete K. Implementation of primary health care: package or process? *SAMJ* 1998; **88**: 1563–65.

[18] WHO. EPI for the 1990s. (WHO/EPI/GEN/92.2, unpublished). Cited in Tarimo E, Webster T. "Primary Health Care Concepts and Challenges in a changing world: Alma Ata revisited." Geneva: WHO, 1994.

[19] The World Bank. *Investing in Health. World Development Report 1993.* Washington DC: The World Bank, 1993.

[20] Hall AJ, Cutts FT. Lessons from measles vaccination in developing countries. *BMJ* 1993; **307**: 1294–5.

[21] Chopra M, Sanders D. Is growth monitoring worthwhile in South Africa? *SAMJ* 1997; **87**: 875–8.

[22] Integrated Regional Information Network. Ethiopia: Campaign to eradicate polio suffers setback, 13 December 2001. Nairobi: UNOCHA, 2001.

[23] Volmink J, Garner P. Systematic review of randomised controlled trials of strategies to promote adherence to tuberculosis treatment. *BMJ* 1997; **315**: 1403–6.

[24] Halstead SB, Walsh JA, Warren K (eds.). *Good Health at Low Cost.* New York: Rockefeller Foundation, 1985.

[25] Fitzroy H, Briend A, Fauveau V. Child survival: Should the strategy be redesigned? Experience from Bangladesh. *Health Pol Planning* 1990; **5**: 226–34.

[26] Janovsky K. The Challenge of Implementation. District Health Systems for Primary Health Care. Geneva: WHO, 1988.

[27] Tarimo E. Towards a healthy district: Organizing and managing district health systems based on primary health care. Geneva: WHO, 1991.

[28] Jeppsson A. Financial priorities under decentralization in Uganda. *Health Pol Planning* 2001; **16**: 187–92.

[29] Breman A, Shelton C. Structural adjustment and health: A literature review of the debate, its role players and the presented empirical evidence. WHO Commission on Macroeconomics and Health Working Paper WG 6:6. Geneva: WHO, 2001.

[30] Bond P. Globalisation, pharmaceutical pricing, and South African health policy: Managing confrontation with U.S. firms and politicians. *Int J Health Services* 1999; **29**: 765–92.

[31] Hong E. Globalisation and the impact on health: A third world view. Third World Network, 2000. Available at http://www.twnside.org.sg/health.htm

[32] See http://www.preamble.org.

[33] SA Business Day, 23 August 2000.

[34] Cassels A. Health Sector Reform: key issues in less developed countries. *J Int Development* 1995; **7**: 338.

[35] Ministry of Health. Medium Term Strategic Framework for Health Development in Ghana 1996–2000. Ghana: MOH, 1995.

[36] WHO-African Regional Office. HR Database, last updated August 2000.

[37] Dovlo DY. Report on Issues affecting the mobility and retention of health workers/professionals in Commonwealth African States. A Consultancy report prepared for the Commonwealth Secretariat, 1999 (Unpublished).

[38] Foster M, Brown A, Norton A, Naschold F. *The Status of Sector Wide Approaches: Centre for Aid and Public Expenditure (CAPE)*. London: ODI, 2000.

[39] Ministry of Health. Independent Review of the Zambian Health Reforms. Volume 1—Main Report. WHO, UNICEF, World Bank, 1996.

[40] Commonwealth Secretariat. *Migration of Health Workers from Commonwealth Countries. Experiences and Recommendations for Action.* London: Commonwealth Secretariat, 2001.

[41] Dovlo D, Nyonator F. Migration of Graduates of the Ghana Medical School: A preliminary rapid appraisal. *Human Resources for Health Dev J* 1999; **3**.

[42] Browne A. Current Issues in Sector-wide Approaches for Health Development—Uganda Case Study. For: Inter-Agency Group on Sector-wide Approaches and Development Cooperation. Geneva: WHO, 2000.

[43] WHO Lesotho Country Team. Health Services in Lesotho: A study of possible cooperation with South Africa. November 1994.

[44] Editorial. The new global health fund. *BMJ* 2001; **322**: 1321–2.

[45] Cassels A. A Guide to sector-wide approaches for health development. Concepts, issues and working arrangements. Geneva: WHO/ARA/97. 12, 1997.

[46] Dubbeldam R., Bijlmakers L. Sector-wide approaches for health development. Dutch experiences in international co-operation. Ministry of Foreign Affairs, the Netherlands, 1999.

[47] Dovlo D, Jonsson U. Personal communication. March 2002.

[48] Verheul E, Rowson M. Poverty reduction strategy papers. It's too soon to say whether this new approach to aid will improve health. *BMJ* 2001; **323**: 120.

[49] WHO, UNICEF. Report of the International Conference on Primary Health Care. Alma-Ata, USSR, 6–12 September 1978.

[50] Sanders D. Success factors in community-based nutrition programmes. *Food and Nutrition Bull* 1999; **20**: 307–14.

[51] Sanders D, Chopra M, Lehmann U, Heywood A. Meeting the Challenge of Health for all through Public Health Education: A Response from the University of the Western Cape. *SAMJ* 2001; **91**: 823–9.

[52] Regional Strategy for the Development of Human Resources for Health. AFR/RC48/10. Harare: WHO Regional Office for Africa, 1998.

[53] Report of the first Multidisciplinary Advisory Group on the development of Human resources for Health, 27–28 March 2000. Harare: WHO Draft Report, 2000.

[54] Mosley H. In: SB Halstead, JA Walsh, K Warren (eds.). *Good Health at Low Cost*. New York: Rockefeller Foundation, 1985.

Chapter 9

Public health in China: History and contemporary challenges

Liming Lee, Vivian Lin, Ruotao Wang and Hongwen Zhao

Introduction

Over the last fifty years China has made great progress in the prevention and control of communicable diseases. This progress is far in excess of what would have been expected at its stage of economic development. Demographic transitions have taken place in most of the cities and economically developed areas in China and the society has evolved from its historical norm in which young people made up the majority to a society with a rapid increase of the middle-aged and elderly populations. In "old China", fertility rates and fatality rates from infectious diseases were high and communicable disease epidemics endangered the health of the entire population, particularly those more vulnerable to disease.

Following the 1949 revolution, safe water supply, sanitation, personal hygiene, together with maternal and child health care became the focus of efforts to improve the health of the population. Over the last few decades as China developed into an aging society, noncommunicable diseases (NCDs) have emerged and behavior-related health problems have prompted an official response. The achievements in public health, however, have been distributed unevenly between urban and rural populations and between economically developed and under-developed areas [1–4].

China now faces serious public health challenges. Environmental pollution has increased. Inequality in the provision of health services has also increased. The maintenance of vaccination programmes and primary health care has become more difficult in poor and remote areas. While the "older infectious diseases" are still threatening people's health in most parts of China, particularly in the economically underdeveloped areas, "newer infectious diseases", such as sexually transmitted diseases (STDs) and HIV, are becoming serious public health problems.

In this chapter, we briefly review the history of public health in China, discuss the achievements of the last fifty years and the emerging problems, analyze the health transition trends, and finally look forward to the prospects for public health in China.

A brief history of public health

Prevention is an integral part of traditional Chinese medicine which considers two aspects of disease states: pathogenic factors and body resistance. In giving priority to strengthening body resistance, conventional wisdom encourages a regular life, a healthy diet, exercise, and harmony in mental and emotional activities.

Western medicine was introduced into China by Christian missionaries in the 1830s. The establishment of the Peking Union Medical College (PUMC) in 1917 by the Rockefeller Foundation provided the framework for educating the new elite of western medicine. In 1921, a public health department was established within PUMC with the aim of providing epidemiological data and a focus for population-based health care [5]. During 1932–37 Professor Chen Zhi-qian (C.C. Chen), a medical graduate of PUMC working in Ding County, established an early example of public health activities integrated with the primary health care system [6].

In 1949, China faced the daunting task of post-war infrastructure reconstruction and a shortage of resources. In the 1950s public health activities in China were dominated by two influences. Firstly, China adopted the public health system of the former Soviet Union, setting up epidemic prevention stations (EPS) all over the country and establishing public health schools separate from medical schools. Secondly, China formed a social movement called the Patriotic Health Campaign Committee (PHCC) to guide the main public health activities, based on experiences during the civil and Korean wars.

The Chinese government set the following guiding principles: focusing on rural areas, giving top priority to prevention, attaching equal importance to traditional medicine and western medicine, mobilizing all sectors of society to participate in health work and serving people's health and the socialist modernization drive. Millions of Chinese were told what they should and should not do in order to improve their health. As a part of the early Patriotic Health Campaign, the government declared a war against "four pests"—flies, mosquitoes, mice, and sparrows. People were instructed to clean their houses, schools and workplaces, as well as to practice personal hygiene techniques every day. The PHCC at national, provincial and city levels, organized inspections to check the implementation of these actions, and to praise people who implemented them well. These campaigns continued throughout the 1960s and 1970s as the dominant form of public health intervention. Together with the "bare-foot doctor" system, established in Chinese rural areas in mid-1960s and during the Cultural Revolution in the 1970s, the PHCC successfully controlled many serious epidemics of communicable diseases, such as cholera, plague, and malaria [7,8].

The organizational frameworks for policy implementation and health services delivery were also influenced by the Soviet Union and still comprise a series of vertical lines: maternal and child health care services (MCH), three-tier healthcare networks (hospitals, health centers, and clinics) in urban and rural areas, and medical colleges (inclusive of public health). Each vertical activity was led by a department within the Ministry of Health (Disease Control, MCH, Medical Administration, and Medical Education, respectively), with services provided at provincial, municipal, county/district, and township/neighborhood levels. In the 1980s, additional agencies were added to the public health infrastructure. The Chinese Academy of Preventive Medicine (CAPM), a technical agency related to the Disease Control Department of the Ministry, and the Centre for Health Statistics and Information (CHSI) are the authoritative sources of public health information.

The public health workforce now comprises mainly graduates from two educational channels, the medical universities and three year secondary medical colleges. The medical university graduates have five to six years of medical and public health training; graduates from three-year secondary medical colleges have vocational training such as MCH care services and epidemic prevention at the community level. Public health doctors are professionally ranked in a similar fashion to those in clinical medicine with three ranks: the senior level placed at city facilities, middle level at county facilities and junior at township level facilities [9].

Core public health activities are delivered by almost 6000 EPS with almost 300,000 technical staff and include: epidemic prevention and infectious disease control, occupational health and safety, environmental health, food hygiene, school health, radiation protection, health inspection, public health laboratory services, and health education [10]. Responsibility for NCD prevention and control was added to the work of the EPS in the mid-1990s. Related primary health care activities, such as

MCH and family planning, have been separately funded, in line with organizational arrangements.

Achievements and challenges

The doubling of life expectancy from thirty-six years in 1950 to seventy-one years in 1998 highlights the Chinese health improvements. In the past fifty years, the population has rapidly expanded in size, increasing from 554 million in the early 1950s to 1259 million in 1999, despite the implementation of the one-child policy. The ratio of "old dependents" (population above age sixty-five as a percentage of the normal working age population, 15–65 years) increased steadily from 7.9 percent in 1980 to 10.3 percent in 2000, and is projected to be almost 20 percent by 2025. In 1999 people over age sixty exceeded 10 percent of the total population. In less than twenty years China transformed from a "young society" to "an elderly one," much faster than Sweden, France and other western developed countries which took 40–150 years to complete this transition. The Chinese population is unique in that it experienced "premature aging" or "aging before getting rich" within a relatively short period of time. This is a great achievement, as well as a challenge from the public health perspective.

The importance of noncommunicable diseases

Since 1949, mortality rates from infectious diseases and conditions affecting maternal and child health, have fallen dramatically. This achievement, together with the rapid population growth, has led to a continuous increase in the burden of NCD [11–13]. Table 9.1 shows the leading causes of death in China. In 2000, NCDs were estimated to account for 61.5 percent of Disability Adjusted Life Years lost (DALYS) in China [14], and Table 9.2 shows the leading causes.

Table 9.1 Leading causes of death as percentage of total deaths, 1999, urban and rural areas

Causes of death	Urban areas (%)	Rural areas (%)
Malignant neoplasms	23.9	18.4
Cerebrovascular disease	21.6	18.4
Respiratory disease	13.9	22.1
Ischaemic heart disease	16.8	12.4
Injury and poisoning	6.3	11.0

Source: Ref. [10].

Table 9.2 Leading causes of DALYs, male and female, 2000

Male	Percent of total	Female	Percent of total
1. Chronic obstructive pulmonary disease	7.7	1. Chronic obstructive pulmonary disease	7.6
2. Cerebrovascular disease	6.0	2. Unipolar depressive disorder	7.1
3. Road traffic accidents	5.0	3. Lower respiratory infections	6.1
4. Unipolar depressive disorders	4.8	4. Cerebrovascular disease	5.4
5. Lower respiratory infections	4.7	5. Perinatal conditions	5.2
6. Perinatal conditions	4.5	6. Self-inflicted injuries	3.6
7. Anaemia	3.3	7. Anaemia	3.4
8. Ischaemic heart disease	3.1	8. Ischaemic heart disease	2.6
9. Falls	2.9	9. Congenital anomalies	2.5
10. Liver cancer	2.7	10. Falls	2.3
All Others	56.4	All Others	54.2

Source: Ref. [15].

Re-emergence of STDs and emergence of HIV

The control of sexually transmitted diseases (STDs) was one of the triumphs of the first public health revolution. STDs began to re-emerge in the early 1980s with the "opening up" of China, although there was no longer a formal reporting system.

The first case of HIV was identified in 1985 and was considered an imported case. It was only a matter of time before an epidemic began. The development of HIV/AIDS in China is characterized by three stages [16]:

(1) from the mid-1980s to 1988, there were sporadic, imported cases amongst foreign travelers in coastal provinces;

(2) from 1989 to 1993, following the identification of 146 HIV positive drug users in Yunnan, there was geographically limited spread;

(3) from 1994 there has been sharp rise among drug users and in sexually-transmitted HIV, and beyond Yunnan to Sichuan (1995), Xinjiang (1996), and Guangxi (1997).

HIV AIDS related to blood transfusion and blood products emerged in the late 1990s as a result of impoverished villagers and migrant workers earning money from blood donation. By September 2001, there were 28,133 HIV positive cases reported and 1208 AIDS patients. During the first half of 2001, the reported HIV positive cases increased 67.4 percent compared to the number reported during the same period the previous year [17]. Two-thirds of these reported HIV positives were infected through sharing syringes/needles used in intravenous drug injections. More than half of the HIV-positive individuals are in their twenties. However, it has been estimated that there were about 600,000 HIV-positive individuals in China at the end of 2000. If no effective interventions take place in China, UNAIDS estimates that there may be as many as six million testing HIV-positive by the year 2005 and more than ten million by the year 2010 [18].

Risk factors for disease

More Chinese are smoking today than ever before and China's cigarette consumption is already the largest in the world. In 1997 the China National Tobacco Corporation was the largest tobacco company in the world, with "Zhong Hua" and "Hong Ta Shan" the leading brands; it produces 25 percent of the total global production. The National Epidemiological Investigation of Smoking and Health in 1996 showed that "the general smoking rate" in the population aged 15+ years was 67 percent for men and four percent for women. It is estimated that in China 300,000 tobacco-related deaths occur per year [19]. Most of these deaths affect the middle-aged population. The burden of tobacco-related illness is likely to increase about 6–10 fold within the next generation and will occur disproportionately in people with less education [20,21].

Dietary change has been rapid in China. In 2000 the "national average daily energy intake" was 2387 calories, 70.5 g of protein, and 54.7 g of fat. Low body weight prevalence in Chinese children under age of five was 19 percent in 1990, but reduced to 11 percent in 2000. However, this nutritional improvement was uneven between urban and rural communities and between economically developed and developing areas. There are three main nutritional problems. Firstly, the so-called "double challenge" exists, that is under-nutrition remains a problem in economically poor areas while an increasing prevalence of obesity appears serious in many cities. Secondly, diseases caused by the shortage of various micronutrients, such as nutritional anemia and iodine deficiency, continue to pose a serious health problem, especially for children. Thirdly, the problem of food safety and hygiene obligates the government to take more effective action in protecting people's health in this area [22].

The Chinese government has for some years recognized the severe health risks posed by environmental pollution. Large-scale efforts in the early 1980s to reduce particulate emissions from heating and power plants have improved air quality in some major cities. However, small industries in rural areas have become serious sources of air pollution. Indoor air pollution from cooking and heating fuels and from volatile substances released in cooking add to the environmental risks in the household, particularly among the poor where wood, dung and soft-coal fuels are frequently used [23,24].

China also faces a serious water crisis with the shortage of water resources and water pollution. Fifty percent of all Chinese cities are short of water. Many rivers and lakes are seriously polluted [22]. Deforestation and loss of soil and fresh-water have led to sand-land spreading at about 2460 sq km annually in recent years. Most importantly, there is not yet effective cooperation between China's National Environmental Protection Agency (NEPA) and the Ministries of Health (MOH), Labor, Industry and other governmental agencies. The NEPA and MOH lack an effective approach for strategy development, monitoring and collaboration, and enforcement of environmental protection policies [21].

Increasing health inequalities

There remain large discrepancies in health status within China between cities and rural areas, and between economically developed areas and developing areas. Most cities and economically developed areas of China have completed "the first health revolution" or "demographic transition." In these areas there is the emerging epidemic of noncommunicable diseases, injuries, and neuro-psychiatric disorders. There is also the persistent problem of infectious diseases and maternal and child health in economically disadvantaged rural and remote parts of China. There are still nearly 100 million Chinese (8 percent of the total population) without health services and safe water and more than thirty million Chinese access health services 5 km away from their home [21]. In 1998, 87 percent of mothers in economically poor areas delivered their babies at home without proper health care, and 13 percent of Chinese children living in economically poor rural areas received no vaccinations [21].

The extent of health and health care inequalities increased over the last twenty years. There is a great disparity in resource distribution between urban and rural areas. About 80 percent of medical resources in China are concentrated in urban areas, two-thirds of which are allocated to big hospitals. Medical services are concentrated in secondary and tertiary hospitals while scant resources are allocated to primary care and rural health services.

Rural health professionals account for only 38 percent of the total health professionals in China, despite the fact that 70 percent of the population lives in the countryside. With escalation of medical care costs at 11–12 percent per annum in the 1990s, the decreasing coverage of health insurance among poor populations, and the increased financial burden on individual and households, there are widespread complaints about access to, and the cost of care, particularly in rural areas. It has been estimated that as many as 50 percent of poor rural households have fallen into poverty because of the cost of health care, with much of that related to catastrophic illnesses, such as NCDs [25,26].

Disaster relief, disease prevention, and bioterrorism

China faces frequent natural disasters, such as floods, droughts, snowstorms, earthquakes, and mud/rock slides. Serious disasters are typically followed by disease epidemics. One great Chinese public health achievement in the last fifty years was the introduction of disaster relief and epidemic prevention programmes. Serious floods occurred along the Yangtze River valleys in southern China in 1954 and 1991, and along the Yangtze, Nenjiang River and Songhua River in 1998; severe earthquakes took place in Xingtai and Tangshan of Hebei Province in 1966 and 1976, respectively. Although no disease epidemics followed these disasters, the response to natural disasters remains one of major public health tasks in China.

Shortly after the terrorist attack on 11 September 2001 in New York, the Chinese government required relevant departments to prepare for possible bioterrorist attacks. The development of rapid response mechanisms for natural disasters and terrorist attacks has become another priority in public health.

Public health responses to the new challenges

The introduction of cost-recovery policies and fiscal decentralization in public administration in the 1980s had adverse impacts on the public health system. Some institutions met their new managerial responsibilities by shifting away from community outreach and preventive services, as the estimated share of government spending on health declined to 15.3 percent by 1999 [10]. The decline in immunization coverage, increase in tuberculosis (TB) occurrence, and the lack of progress in infant and maternal mortality rates have been attributed to these developments [25].

Health reform has attracted much attention recently in Chinese politics and the community at large. The State Council issued a decision on health reform in 1997, established basic health insurance for employees in the cities in 1998, and made further suggestions for health reform in cities in early 2000. A major national workshop was held in 2000 to discuss Health Strategy Reform and Development [21]. The landmark 1997 State Council paper on Health Development and Reform [27] requested all levels of government to provide full budgetary support to public health institutions and to halt inappropriate practices related to the introduction of market incentives.

The implementation of these directives has been uneven. The policy framework has been further translated into priorities for the MOH in the Tenth Five-Year Plan (2001–2005). The priorities are:

+ rural health reforms including basic health services and cooperative medical service (CMS) development;

+ health sector reform, including regional health planning, hospital management reforms, sale and management of pharmaceuticals, and community health services development;

+ reform of health inspection;

+ control of new and re-emerging diseases, including HIV/STD, NCD and TB.

The priorities in a five-year plan, however, do not necessarily reflect the day-to-day preoccupation of health administrators. The reform programme adopted in 2000 is more suggestive of the day-to-day priorities, particularly the preoccupation with hospitals and health financing issues. The new focus is on urban health insurance, regulating urban hospitals, drug price and dispensing reforms, and personnel reforms. In this context, public health oriented reforms (such as community health service development and health inspection reforms) are less likely to receive high-level attention.

China's entry into the World Trade Organization in 2001 poses new challenges for public health practice, for example, the reduction in tariffs on imported tobacco products. Government health authorities are conducting reviews to consider which areas of internal regulation practice will have to be abandoned, which areas of work will be de-regulated, and which areas will require strengthening of regulations.

Foundations for the future

The original NCD control efforts, starting in the 1980s, were focused on treatment of particular diseases, in the same way that earlier infectious disease control efforts were targeted at particular diseases. Similarly, the early efforts on HIV prevention and control adopted the traditional disease control paradigm. Because of the small scope of community-based interventions and the sporadic nature of the health education activities, discussions about NCD or STD/HIV control have been dominated by a medical management or case management approach. Some prominent, retired clinicians and public health academics and officials are now mobilizing public attention around the NCD and HIV epidemics, initiating community prevention programmes and championing the newly approved NGOs dedicated to the cause of HIV prevention and control.

Lessons from NCD prevention programme

The major NCD prevention programme of the 1990s introduced health promotion concepts and methods through a combined approach to intervening on key risk factors (smoking, nutrition, physical activity, hypertension) and in key settings (schools, workplaces, neighborhoods) in seven cities. These cities have enacted and enforced a range of tobacco control regulations, as well as pioneering ventures for regulations and policies in other areas, including salt labeling, health education curriculum in schools, and hypertension management in hospitals. Many programme models are successful in pilot areas, such as nutritious lunch in schools, health quiz shows on television, diabetes clubs, nonsmoking families/shops/workplaces, "quit and win" competitions, and community physical activity facilities. Data over four years from the behavioral risk factor surveillance system demonstrate the positive impact of the project in raising awareness about tobacco, hypertension, nutrition, and other lifestyle risk factors [28].

This proactive approach to health promotion requires supportive regulatory and legislative actions. This is more a political issue than a technical one; for example, there is still argument as to whether tobacco production should generate more profits and national revenues, or whether more should be done to prevent the millions of Chinese expected to die from tobacco-related illness by the year 2025 [1]. The need for policy action is particularly important, given weak public efforts to intervene on lifestyle risk factors and the strong presence of increasing and powerful private enterprises. Insofar as many of the determinants of health behavior will require interventions from outside the health sector, such as education and agriculture, developing a genuinely multi-sectoral response to NCDs remains a major policy challenge.

Experiences from HIV/AIDS prevention and control

The initial national response was to create an institutional framework for AIDS prevention and control focused on the health sector [29]. A National AIDS Committee was set up in 1986, a national AIDS Prevention and

Control Programme developed in 1987, a MOH Medium-term Plan issued in 1990, and the Chinese Association of STD/AIDS Prevention and Control (a government-sponsored NGO) was established in 1992. During the early period, the priority was on keeping HIV/AIDS out of China and providing a traditional public health infectious disease surveillance response. Laws and regulations were enacted on "frontier health and quarantine", prohibition of narcotic drugs and prostitution, and for surveillance and testing in select population groups as well as case reporting. The information infrastructure includes 100 sentinel sites for six populations, ad hoc surveys (including sero- and behavioral surveys), and thirty-six laboratories.

China responded to the HIV epidemic with an initial focus on surveillance. Other strategies emerged gradually during the 1990s. For instance, in the mid-1990s public sector STD clinics did not provide anonymous treatment, gave limited attention to privacy and confidentiality, and charged large fees for clinical consultation, laboratory confirmation, and prophylaxis. A burgeoning private sector of unregulated clinics failed to diagnose and treat properly. By the end of the 1990s, management of public clinics began to shift to syndromic treatment, anonymous treatment, and respecting privacy and confidentiality, and condoms and patient education became available [30].

In 1996, the Government became more concerned and established a State Council AIDS Coordinating Committee (involving thirty-three ministries and mass organizations). A joint MOH and UNAIDS report in 1997 set out the strategic directions for development. In 1998, an AIDS Expert Committee was formed and the State Council released its medium and long-term Plan, signaling serious commitment to action. Much of the concern in the second half of the 1990s was prompted by reports about contamination of blood products and blood supply, as can be seen in the major legislative responses in 1996 (Regulation on management of blood donation) and 1998 (Law on Blood Donation). A broader public health approach was finally introduced into policy in 1998, when the Government issued Principles for HIV Education and Communication. Following collaboration with multiple international organizations and exposure to a wide array of contemporary public health practices in a range of countries, by the late 1990s there were noticeable changes in the approaches being adopted within China. The didactic teaching approach was shifting towards a health promotion approach. Multiple strategies were adopted to work at the policy, community, group, and individual levels. Condom social marketing, youth peer education, training of mass media, integration of HIV into reproductive health services, harm reduction for drug users, strategic planning, sexuality education, workplace projects, creative use of traditional and modern media, and community outreach for vulnerable populations can all be found in China.

The Chinese response to the HIV epidemic is poised to confront the magnitude of the challenge. The earlier policy panic may be shifting to genuine multi-sectoral mobilization. The social and economic impact of the HIV epidemic are being quantified. While the underlying dynamic of poverty, migration, and gender roles is complex, new development priorities on poverty alleviation, particularly in Western China, may address some of the fundamental issues behind the epidemic.

Institutional reform: Chinese Center for Disease Control and Prevention

The National Center for Disease Control and Prevention was established in January 2002. This is the first time China has had an agency at the national level for disease control and prevention. The Center has specific responsibility for policy analysis and implementation, information and surveillance, priority setting and management, operational research, and professional training.

Although there are over 400 medical research institutes in China that can investigate the aetiology of and treatment for diseases, it will be the network of EPS that will serve as the foundation for supporting the public health approach to the challenges of the twenty-first century. The function of EPS is, traditionally, to prevent infectious diseases (including the new challenge of HIV); current reforms have directed that their role be broadened to include NCDs, including health promotion. They will, however, need to work out their roles in relation to another new policy development, community health services [31].

The EPS are being transformed into local centers for disease control and prevention. Whether this reform will result in an improved public health infrastructure and capacity will depend, in part, on adequate financing and accountability systems. There is a need for a budgetary framework that supports a coordinated approach to public health activities. There is also a need for a clear legislative framework for operational activities and a shift away from user pays toward full public funding for salaries and operating costs. The public health workforce needs to adopt contemporary public health practices.

Rural health security and regional health planning

The rural three-tier health and disease prevention networks that used to be a source of pride have collapsed in most regions as a consequence of economic reforms. Approximately 85 percent of the population have to pay for health services from their own pockets, and many families fall into poverty as a consequence of health care costs. Rural health workers are technically less competent as a whole, and village doctors are unable to satisfy health care needs. As a result of the tremendous efforts over many years, a relatively complete service and management system for childhood immunization has been established, but financial and technical difficulties may impede the further development of these programmes.

Some regions have experimented with prepayment systems for immunization and MCH services. Others have introduced medical financial assistance schemes for the very poor. Attempts to re-establish CMS have been difficult to sustain, particularly in poor areas [32]. There is an urgent need for social assurance programs, including health insurance, for the most needy, including socially marginalized groups. Restoring and developing the rural three-tier health and disease prevention networks will be important in the battle against the health inequalities between urban and rural areas in China.

The policy of "regional health planning" needs to be fully implemented so that health resources are allocated according to the health needs of all residents in a region. Structural reforms needed in the Chinese health system include: investing in effective health promotion programs; increasing public funding for areas with great need; and continuing to restructure existing medical and health services to effect a system that is community-based, public health oriented, low cost, and responsive to the needs of the local population.

Public health information resource system

Currently there are many disease surveillance systems and various epidemiological data in China. One is the communicable disease reporting system. Key communicable diseases are legally required to be reported monthly; some of the twenty-five key diseases require immediate reporting by phone. Because chronic diseases have emerged as an important problem throughout China, a reporting system has also been established for them, but it is not yet as comprehensive or systematic as that employed for communicable diseases. Routine surveillance data are based on a variety of information about hospital in-patients and out-patients, as part of reporting by hospitals and other health care institutions to the local health bureaux. The maternal and child health care services, endemic diseases control departments and other authorities maintain specialized diseases reporting systems. In the 1980s a system called Disease Surveillance Points (DSP) was established. The DSP system was extended to cover 100 points in 1989 and is being modified to provide better quality data on a stratified, random sample of China's urban and rural population.

Unfortunately the current disease surveillance system fails to report epidemics in a timely and accurate manner, which leads to a delayed response to epidemics across China. Epidemiologists at all levels are unable to use the current information system to improve their research. Medical care workers are also unable to use the information to keep their services up-to-date. The current disease surveillance system in China fails to provide enough information for health policy analysis and decision making. This system also fails to provide useful information for health law and policy evaluation and fails to support effective health education and communication activities. These reporting systems are undergoing reform and consolidation. More importantly, disease surveillance systems should be expanded to be a public health information resource system—a broad information collection and exchange system in public health. This system should collect and consolidate all relevant information to serve health policy analysis and decision making, to provide necessary information for effective health communication and education, and to supply useful knowledge for epidemiologists and other health care professionals. This system could also provide a forum for an open participatory discussion with communities about major public health issues.

Conclusion

China has achieved great successes in public health in the past fifty years. However, China faces even more serious challenges in the future. Among these challenges are the control of NCD and HIV/AIDS and the battle for healthy environments and equity in health. These new priorities require policy and infrastructure reforms in health as well as multi-sectoral co-operation, including with NGOs and private health enterprises. China is actively drawing lessons from other countries in pursuit of a path that is suited to local conditions. The newly established Chinese Center for Disease Control and Prevention will play an important role in shaping the future of public health in China.

The rapid economic development over the past twenty years, the accelerated pace of industrialization and urbanization, and the widening of the income gap between population groups, will determine the current and future health needs among individuals and communities. A sustainable and successful approach to addressing these major challenges will require the incorporation of the underlying social, cultural, and economic factors into public health interventions. Creating an enabling environment, including regulatory and legal system development, and complementary policies in such sectors as agriculture and education will also be needed. A paradigm shift in public health practice will need to start with developing a critical mass of public health professionals equipped with new knowledge and skills.

Cautious optimism remains for the development of public health in China in the near future. Insofar as China continues to strive for new approaches to handle new challenges, it will continue to offer lessons for other countries.

Acknowledgement

We thank Prue Bagley for research and editorial assistance and Chen Jie for helpful comments.

References

[1] World Bank. China: Long-Term Issues and Options in the Health Transition. Washington, DC: World Bank, 1992.

[2] Chen X, Hu T, Lin Z. The rise and decline of the cooperative medical system in rural China. *Int J Health Services* 1993; **23**: 731–42.

[3] Hsiao W. The Chinese Health Care System: Lessons for other nations. *Soc Sci Med* 1995; **41**: 1047–55.

[4] Beaglehole R, Bonita R. *Public Health at the Crossroads*. Oxford: Oxford University Press, 1997.

[5] Brown ER. *Rockefeller Medicine Men: Medicine and Capitalism in America*. Berkeley: University of California Press, 1979.

[6] Chen Z. *Medicine in Rural China—A personal Account*. Chengdu: Sichuan People's Press, 1997.

[7] Wang R. Critical health literacy: a case study from China in schistosomiasis control. *Hth Promot Int* 2000; **15**: 269–74.

[8] Horn J. *Away with All Pests*. New York: Monthly Review Press, 1969.

[9] Lee L. Facing the Challenges of the 21st Century Professional education in Public Health in China, Paper presented at "Issues and Challenges of Public Health in the 21st century (New Millenium Series)", University of Malaysia, 1996.

[10] Ministry of Health. Chinese Health Statistical Digest. Beijing: Ministry of Health, 2000.

[11] Li X, Deng S. Some aspects of diabetes care in Chengdu. *Soc Sci Med* 1995; **41**: 1185–90.

[12] Chen Z, Xu Z, Collins R et al. Early health effects of the emerging tobacco epidemic in China: A 1—year prospective study. *JAMA* 1997; **278**: 1500–4.

[13] Pan X, Yang W, Li G, Juang L. Prevalence of diabetes and its risk factors in China 1994. *Diabetes Care* 1997; **20**: 1664–72.

[14] Murray CL, Lopez AD. *The Global Burden of Disease and Injury Series*, Vol. 1. Cambridge: Harvard University Press, 1996.

[15] Murray CJL, Lopez AD, Mathers CD, Stein C. The Global Burden of Disease 2000 project: aims, methods and data sources. Geneva, World Health Organization, 2000 (GPE Discussion Paper No. 36), 2001. (www.who.int/evidence)

[16] Ministry of Health, UN Theme Group on HIV/AIDS in China. China Responds to AIDS. Beijing: Ministry of Health, 1997.

[17] Zhang W. Speech at the First Chinese Conference on AIDS/STD Control. Beijing, November 2001.

[18] UNAIDS. China Update. 2000.

[19] *Smoking and Health in China—1996 National Prevalence Survey of Smoking Pattern*. Beijing: Science-technology Press, 1997.

[20] Yang G, Fan L, Tan J et al. Smoking in China: Findings of the 1996 national prevalence survey. *JAMA* 1999; **282**: 1247–53.

[21] Yu Z, Nissinen A, Vartiainen E *et al.* Associations between socioeconomic status and cardiovascular risk factors in an urban population in China. *Bull WHO* 2000; **78**: 1296–1305.

[22] Document of High-level Forum for Public Nutrition and Social-economic Development. Beijing, December 2001.

[23] Monographs for Health Reform and Development Strategy Workshop. Internal communication. Beijing, June 2000.

[24] Liu Q, Sasco A, Riboli E, Meng XH. Indoor Air Pollution and Lung Cancer in Guangzhou, People's Republic of China. *Am J Epidemiol* 1993; **137**: 145–54.

[25] World Bank. China: Financing Health Care. Washington, DC: World Bank, 1997.

[26] China Health Economics Institute, Institute for Development Studies. Proceedings from the Conference on China Rural Health Reform and Development. Beijing: China Health Economic Institute (CHEI) and Institute of Development Studies (IDS), 2000.

[27] State Council. Decision on Health Reform and Development. Beijing, January 1997.

[28] Presentation by Chinese Academy of Preventive Medicine at Disease Prevention (Health Promotion) Project Supervision. Chengdu, April 2000.

[29] Ministry of Health and UN Theme Group on HIV/AIDS in China. China Responds to AIDS. Beijing: Ministry of Health, 1997.

[30] Jiang T. Social and Economic Impact of HIV/AIDS in Guangdong. Paper presented at the 6th International Congress on AIDS in Asia and the Pacific, Melbourne, October 2001.

[31] Ministry of Health. Research on National Health Services—An Analysis Report of the 2nd National Health Services Survey in 1998, Volume I. Beijing: MOH, 1998.

[32] Yu H, Lucas H, Gu X, Shu B. Financing Health Care in Poor Rural Counties in China: experience from a township-based co-operative medical scheme. Sussex: IDS working paper 66, 1998; Carrin G, Ron A, Yang H et al. The reform of the rural cooperative medical system in the People's Republic of China: interim experience in 14 pilot counties, *Soc Sci Med* 1999; **48**: 961–72.

Chapter 10

Public health in South Asia

T Jacob John and Franklin White

Introduction

South Asian countries (Bangladesh, Bhutan, India, Maldives, Nepal, Pakistan, Sri Lanka) share a rich heritage. Once the cradle of ancient Indus Valley and Dravidian civilizations, over centuries the social fabric was enriched by immigration from diverse sources. Today the region is a kaleidoscope of ethnic, linguistic, religious and political entities, with strong cultural and behavioral similarities, all of which influence "public health". Low levels of income and literacy and heavy burdens of disease characterize much of the region.

Several systems of medicine are widely practiced in the region. The ancient "Ayurveda" system ranged from magico-mythical to the physical and the rational. Its pharmacopoeia of herbal and plant products is enormous. "Siddha", a related system using heavy metals, is popular in southern India. "Unani", adopted from Arabian medicine, is popular in northern regions, while homeopathy is practiced everywhere. Faith healers abound, while folk practitioners treat broken bones and conditions ranging from paralytic illnesses to snakebite. Since British colonial rule, "modern" medicine ("allopathy") was adopted as the official system by governments throughout the region. In the indigenous systems, disease is perceived to be due to imbalance between internal "principles" within the body; infectious diseases are recognized and treated but, microbes generally are not understood as causal agents. Modern "public health" concepts did not develop within any indigenous system, although healthy habits emphasizing dietary rules, body cleanliness, meditation and yoga, are integral to some systems.

The British introduced elementary public health programs during the nineteenth and early twentieth centuries. Although the health of the rulers was more important than that of the ruled, the lack of public health development during half a century of independence can no longer be blamed on colonial rule. Many believe that diseases and their cure are determined by external influences (deities, planetary/stellar configurations, evil spirits) or by predestination [1]. As microbial causation is not understood by many people, cleanliness often has only a symbolic or ritualistic meaning. For example, water being a cleansing agent, how can it not be clean? It is not uncommon for a water source to be used (simultaneously) for bathing, drinking, ablution after defecation, laundry and washing buffaloes. As in wealthier countries, the educated, including physicians, teachers and policy makers are more attracted to curative medicine than prevention, partly due to the ready availability of drugs. Fundamental public health applications of medical science (clean water, sanitation, hygiene education) have still to be fully implemented. This problem is reflected in the current response to the emergence of noncommunicable disease, focusing on individual diagnosis and treatment rather than primary prevention and public health interventions.

All South Asian countries are improving their health status through family planning, training of birth attendants, immunization, popularization of oral hydration for diarrhoea, and enabling private sector medical care. However, there is still a need to use public health measures to impact more directly on the underlying determinants of disease burden [2,3]. For example, Kerala state in India, often cited, along with Sri Lanka, as a model for achieving "good health status at low cost," [4] is endemic for diseases associated with poor environmental conditions. The number of persons per 1000 reporting acute ailments during fifteen day periods was eighty-eight and sixty-one in rural and urban Kerala, against national averages of forty-five and forty-one, respectively, while for chronic ailments, the rates were thirty-eight and twenty-seven, against national averages of thirteen and fourteen [5]. District level surveillance in Kerala showed that by far the commonest diseases reported are acute dysenteries, typhoid fever and leptospirosis [6]. While Sri Lanka has the highest overall health status in the region, it also remains endemic for conditions associated with poor environments. More generally, the focus in South Asia on improving summary indicators of population health (e.g., fertility, infant mortality, life expectancy), and on the provision of costly medical care, has obscured a large burden of infectious diseases, malnutrition and other preventable conditions, and their determinants.

Population, human development and health status

South Asian countries vary widely. India with three-quarters of the land area and population has enormous diversity in health status with the southern states being outstanding performers. Maldives, by contrast, is an archipelago of fewer than a half million people. Sri Lanka and the Maldives, both island states, lead the region on the United Nations Human Development Index (ranked eighty-fourth and eighty-ninth, respectively), while the others lag considerably. Except for Sri Lanka, there is an excess of males, reflecting the magnitude of the disadvantage of being female throughout most of the region. Taking into account data availability, we selected four countries for closer comparison: Sri Lanka, India, Bangladesh and Pakistan (Table 10.1).

In terms of epidemiological transition theory, Sri Lanka and the Maldives fit the rapid transitional variant, reflecting faster socio-economic development, while the other countries are in slow transition [10]. Mortality in the former was declining by the mid-twentieth century, followed by a rapid decline in fertility. The other countries showed later mortality declines with fertility falling only slowly, and now experience considerable burdens of communicable and nutritional diseases, with a recent rise in noncommunicable diseases (NCDs). In disadvantaged areas more epidemiological "accumulation" than transition may be taking place. Despite pockets of development, the general situation is of relative stagnation, compounded by poor governance, corruption, and low investment in economic and social development. Only Sri Lanka is characterized by high literacy and relative gender equality. The other countries exhibit minimal investment on health, education and technology, and relatively closed economies. All countries in the region have incurred large foreign debt burdens and, as with many other countries, allocate more to military expenditures than to health.

The most preventable health problems affect women and children, reflecting their low status and inadequate social and educational opportunities. Pakistan (total fertility rate (TFR) 5.6) shows the least favorable fertility

Table 10.1 Key indicators of population health and development [7–9]

Country	Population (millions)	Life expectancy at birth (years)			Literacy		Human Development Index (HDI)	Rank (HDI)	Sex ratio (males per 100 females)
		Total	Male	Female	Female	Male			
Bangladesh	133.5	59	59	59	24	48	0.46	146	104.9
India	1033.0	61	60	61	35	64	0.56	128	106.7
Pakistan	145.0	60	60	61	22	48	0.52	135	106.6
Sri Lanka	19.5	72	70	74	86	93	0.73	84	97.8

trends, India and Bangladesh have shown more rapid declines (currently TFR 3.2 and 3.3, respectively), while Sri Lanka has achieved stability (2.1, or "zero growth") [7]. Bangladesh and Pakistan warrant closer comparison, given their common political origins following partition from India. The former successfully focused on raising contraceptive prevalence; family planning programs in Pakistan were less successful, mainly due to inconsistent political support. Modern contraceptive methods are now used by >40 percent of women in Sri Lanka, India and Bangladesh, while this is true for <15 percent of Pakistani women [7]. Pregnancy itself is hazardous throughout the subcontinent, due to poor antenatal care and unsafe deliveries, the latter reflected in high maternal mortality ratios (MMR, maternal deaths per 100,000 live births). In 2001 WHO, UNICEF and UNFPA estimated an MMR of 430 for South Asia, while it is only twelve in industrialized countries). Although MMR is an unreliable measure [11], Bangladesh has the most dangerous situation, followed by India and Pakistan; again, Sri Lanka does better.

The high MMR on the subcontinent is due to delay in recognition of risk at home, delay in communications and transportation, and delay in accessing emergency obstetric care following arrival at a hospital [12]. Few women receive care from a provider trained in midwifery, the critical determinant of pregnancy outcome (Bangladesh 4 percent, Pakistan 19 percent, and India 34 percent) [13]. By contrast, 94 percent of Sri Lankan women and a similar proportion of women in Kerala receive such care. The role of traditional birth attendants in the three high risk countries is controversial: can they be trained to become safe and effective in settings where few alternatives exist, especially given that most high risk deliveries occur among ostensibly low risk women? [14]

Infant and child mortality are improving only slowly. The Infant Mortality Rates (IMR) for Bangladesh and India (fifty-eight and seventy per 1000 live births, respectively) reflect those of developing countries generally; Pakistan (IMR 84) trails, while Sri Lanka (IMR 17) contrasts favourably [7]. Child (<5 year) mortality rates (per 1000) show a similar pattern (Bangladesh 89, India 98, Pakistan 112, Sri Lanka 19). Except for Sri Lanka, both measures incorporate high neonatal mortality. Childhood deaths are mostly due to diarrhoea, malnutrition, respiratory infections and vaccine preventable diseases. Due to a combination of traditional birth practices and inadequate maternal immunization, India and Pakistan rank first and third in the world for neonatal tetanus, and four of ten children are "missed opportunities for routine immunizations". [15–17] Although oral rehydration therapy (ORT) is promoted, every second South Asian child with diarrhoea does not receive ORT [17]. The underlying problems of unsafe water, inadequate sanitation, poor food handling practices, and low levels of personal hygiene, persist throughout the region.

In terms of overall disease burden, the estimated trends for India are perhaps most indicative for South Asia as a whole: the Global Burden of Disease study (1996) projects a major shift in disease between 1990 and 2020, from 50.5 percent to 24.4 percent of DALYs (disability adjusted life years) attributable to communicable diseases, from 40.4 percent to 56.5 percent for NCDs, and from 9.1 to 19.1 percent for injuries [18]. Communicable diseases (CDs) continue to pose a major burden, particularly among the poor and contribute to the increasing burden of some cancers. In addition to childhood diseases, the persistence of tuberculosis, malaria and typhoid fever, and the emergence of drug resistant strains, are major concerns [19–21]. Hepatitis (B and C) is hyperendemic, partly due to widespread unsafe injection practices [22]. The potential for HIV transmission is related to proximity to endemic areas both between and within countries; travel and other behaviors conducive to transmission (e.g., increasing injecting drug use) render regional dissemination inevitable. The current HIV situation varies and the data are sparse. It appears that in India HIV infection is widespread and spreading, but in Pakistan only high risk groups are affected (a "high risk low prevalence" country) [23–25]. Similarly, Bangladesh appears to have a relatively low prevalence of sexually transmitted infections [26]. However, other more common reproductive tract infections also need attention, particularly bacterial vaginosis which is linked to adverse perinatal outcomes, and may offer new avenues for intervention [26,27].

As a result of population ageing and socio-behavioral changes associated with urbanization, NCDs are now epidemic in the four countries. In numerous studies internationally, South Asians show a higher incidence and worse outcomes from NCDs than most other populations [28]. Maternal undernutrition leading to impaired organogenesis during fetal development, may play an underlying role, compounded by ongoing suboptimal nutrition [29]. Diabetes prevalence rates are higher than in North America or western Europe. India leads the world in total caseload, while Pakistan (eighth in 1995) is expected to move into fourth position by 2025 [30]. For the region, a 3-fold increase in diabetes caseload is projected by 2025, while the expected increase in the prevalence of hypertension (now affecting one in five adults) is almost as steep [31]. These upswings are propelling an increase in debilitating complications (e.g., renal failure and stroke). National data on circulatory disease risk factors are not available for India. Pakistan's National Health Survey estimated prevalences for adults of: smoking 23 percent (males 34 percent, females 12.5 percent), hypertension 17.9 percent, diabetes 11 percent, and dyslipidemia 12.6 percent [32]. Overweight and obesity are increasing: body mass index is higher in urban than rural areas for all age-sex groups [32]. Given the context of fetal and early childhood malnutrition, the lifestyle changes (diet, physical activity) encountered among urbanizing adults portend large future NCD burdens across the socioeconomic spectrum. Effective and affordable preventive strategies are urgently required [33]. Encouragement may be taken from neighboring countries: Mauritius demonstrated a favorable impact of policy interventions on NCD risk factors, and a study in da Qing, China, showed that the incidence of type two diabetes declined substantially following diet and exercise interventions [34,35]. Developing such policy and lifestyle intervention models is essential, as purely clinical interventions are not affordable for most people or governments. However, in South Asian countries the incorporation of NCD prevention programs within health policy, primary health care or public health generally, has not yet occurred.

The broader agenda of public health remains undeveloped, for example, there are few programs for mental health issues, especially anxiety and depression among women, which are sometimes linked with domestic violence [36]. Son preference underlies a spectrum of issues [37]. Amartya Sen drew attention to "more than 100 million missing women". [38] Most of this gap relates to differential neglect, excess mortality and abortion secondary to prenatal sex selection. More extreme actions such as selective infanticide, "honor killings" and "dowry killings" still occur, although their extent has not been estimated. Child labour is highly prevalent with associated health impacts [39]. Toxic exposures (e.g., to lead and pesticides) are pervasive, reflecting poor environmental controls and inadequate occupational hygiene [40]. Tobacco marketing is targeting youth, compounding other substance abuse (e.g., betel nuts and paan, associated with oral cancers) [41]. Injuries are increasing, especially among young adult males [42]. There are threats to social stability that can be resolved only through developing avenues for dialogue and conflict management. Flashpoints exist within and between countries, having roots in religious intolerance and discrimination by tribe, race and caste, or simple disregard for human impacts (e.g., population displacement following water diversion projects). Vulnerability is widespread, especially for refugees. The only forum for intercountry coordination of development, health and social policies, the South Asian Association for Regional Cooperation (SAARC), is more often a victim of regional politics than a solution to its problems. Health and peace requires that priority be given to human development, especially literacy and gender equity, and sound public health initiatives.

"Health for all" in South Asia

While industrialized nations controlled many CDs in part through public health action addressing transmission channels, low income countries continue to suffer heavy burdens from these diseases. In view of this problem, decentralized control of locally prevalent diseases was proposed within "Primary Health Care" (PHC), a strategy to achieve the visionary, but romanticized, goal of "Health For All" (by 2000). This goal and PHC were declared and defined in 1978 at the famous Alma Ata World Conference, under the aegis of the World Health Organization (WHO) and the United Nations Children's Fund (UNICEF), where 134 countries were represented [43]. Components of PHC included nutritional adequacy, safe water, sanitation, maternal and child health, immunization, medical care for common illnesses (including access to essential drugs), control of locally prevalent diseases and community level "health education". This list blended medical and public health elements. The importance of medical care was widely appreciated. Public health, however, was less understood, especially methods of implementing comprehensive public health programs.

If a higher priority had been given to promoting leadership skills, developing countries might have acquired the self-reliance to progress both in public health and in making basic medical care accessible, particularly to rural and disadvantaged populations. Interestingly, this did not happen. In 1979, the year after the Alma Ata declaration, a group of global experts questioned the feasibility of PHC, and started a counter movement, curiously named "selective PHC" as an interim strategy for disease control in developing countries [44]. The principle of selective PHC was to apply, in a centralized or vertical fashion, using modern analytical and technical tools, skills and knowledge to control infectious diseases, selected from a global list of twenty-three [45]. Over the next few years, WHO itself accepted "selective PHC", and its Director General even wrote the Foreword for the book that crystallized this approach [45]. No doubt, both these approaches, the decentralized, capacity building model of PHC and the centralized, specific and goal-oriented selective disease control approach, were genuine attempts to reintroduce public health to developing country Health Ministries. However, the contradictory elements confused countries. While nearly all had agreed on PHC, WHO approval and donor funding were easier for selective initiatives. The ensuing two decades witnessed at least partial failure of both approaches. Either way, public health was the casualty, and no less in South Asia.

The WHO now questions the very basis of "Primary Health Care", stating: "Despite its many virtues, a criticism of this route (PHC as a route to achieve health for all) has been that it gave too little attention to people's demand for health care ..." [46]. To remedy this, a "new universalism" is advocated, to deliver high quality essential care, defined by criteria of effectiveness, cost and social acceptability. While no one will argue against medical care, the lack of attention to more fundamental public health measures by WHO is cause for concern.

Progress and pitfalls in selective disease control

Despite these policy conflicts, successes have occurred. For example, in 1993 Pakistan searching village by village, treating cases on the spot, providing health education and water supply improvements, was the first country to eliminate Guinea worm infection (GWI) which had been endemic during the 1980s [47]. India reported its first GWI-free year in 1997 [48]. Pending certification, the whole of South Asia may now be disease free. Iodine deficiency has received attention throughout the region and progress has been made implementing iodized salt programs; surveys in Bhutan and New Delhi reveal that these programs are still incomplete [49]. On the environmental front, the Government of India phased out lead as an additive in automotive fuel, and this should steadily restore the cognitive development of children by removing this source of brain toxicity [40]. Similar measures are now advocated in other countries. These and other examples demonstrate that selective interventions can succeed in South Asia.

Nonetheless, there is a "down side". The success of the global eradication of smallpox, through an unprecedented strategy of maintaining "the reproductive rate of infection" [50] below one by surveillance to detect chains of transmission and vaccination to intercept them, had ushered in a new paradigm of global vertical programs. It was in this climate that the experts who reflected on policies on behalf of developing countries unilaterally rerouted the journey towards "health for all" to selective disease control. Thus, nationwide, vertical, single disease control programs against tuberculosis, leprosy, malaria, polio, measles and lymphatic filariasis (and HIV/AIDS in the 1990s) were launched, endorsed by WHO and financed by external donors. Countries learned that selective programs get funding, but with little incentive to integrate them within a broader base of public health programming. However, vertical programs against every important disease is not feasible; the burden of diseases not in the vertical programs remains high and these diseases do not receive appropriate public attention, control activities or adequate funding. Until integrated disease prevention and control models are developed, we will continue to falter in dealing with priorities such as tuberculosis and malaria, let alone meet the complex NCD challenge that is part of the "double burden" of communicable and NCD.

From the UN charter to the peoples health assembly

Health is enshrined in the UN charter of Human Rights and increasingly in national constitutions. However, injustices related to the "globalization" of trade and commerce more generally, are now contributing to ill health and an inability to redress it. Unless this force is balanced with good governance and decentralized decision-making, the health of the poor may be further adversely affected. It is a basic tenant of public health that, in addition to human behavior, external factors (physical, social, political and economic) strongly impact on health, and that interventions must therefore consider all relevant influences. Such sentiments were articulated by a People's Health Assembly convened in Dhaka in 2000. The Assembly attracted delegates from 113 countries, and formulated a *People's Charter of Health*. The Charter expresses disappointment over the unrealized goal of "health for all", which was distorted and disowned by major international players. Like Alma Ata in 1978, this new Charter encourages policy reflections *by the people* instead of *on behalf of the people*. The principal demand is "Health for All, Now", through PHC and appropriate public health programs, emphasizing the social and economic roots of ill health and poverty, and their mutual linkages; fundamentally, it calls for a health paradigm shift from a biomedical to a socioeconomic perspective [51].

The health system

District level health systems exist throughout the region with variations by country. Typically under a District Health Officer or Medical Officer of Health (MOH), there is usually responsibility for district hospitals. Local level dispensaries report to health centres which refer in turn to subdistrict hospitals and so on. The progression is from simple to more complex organizations. In remote villages, a dispensary may be staffed by health visitors who manage common ailments and supply health education. As one ascends the hierarchy, the professional depth and diversity increases, as does the capacity to conduct tests and procedures. This system is intended to integrate curative medicine and public health at community level, consistent with the Alma Ata vision. However, the major problem is that the leadership at most levels is inadequately trained in epidemiology and public health. For example, internists, obstetricians or even surgeons are often posted as MOHs on a seniority basis with administration as their main job. Paradoxically physicians with higher education in public health are posted to run emergency rooms in hospitals, or to other services for which they are not trained. As a result of this human resource mismanagement, there has been a relative lack of coherent public health career advancement opportunities based on relevant training, competence and merit; the salaries and status of public health practitioners remain low.

While all countries have such hierarchical systems in place, critical PHC components have failed to develop. Most physicians appointed to these posts (including many involved in policy decisions) lacked relevant training. It was unrealistic to entrust this system with measures such as provision of safe water, sanitation and vector control, or the community development initiatives required to foster the participatory approach anticipated by Alma Ata, let alone the intersectoral and marketing skills to address contemporary issues such as the emergence of NCDs. The system has done reasonably well on childhood immunization and (in some areas) family planning, when led by physicians untrained in epidemiology and disease control. However, PHC health centres all too often have not succeeded in developing functional surveillance systems to identify or investigate locally prevalent diseases.

Attempts to reintroduce public health into the health system

India is often taken as a "bellweather" from which lessons may be derived for South Asia as a whole. In 1994 a small outbreak of plague occurred in Gujarat state. The public scare created by an unprepared health system, compounded by inaccurate news reporting and over-reaction by public health agencies in some western countries, resulted in major disruptions to international travel and trade, ultimately causing national economic losses of approximately two billion US dollars [52]. It is of interest that another plague outbreak in 2002 produced no major reaction [53].

In response to the 1994 outbreak the Government of India appointed a Technical Advisory Committee on Plague, which identified the national need for trained epidemiologists and pointed out the dearth of training institutions [54]. An Expert Committee on Public Health System in 1996 recommended: articulation of a contemporary national health policy, a modern Public Health Act, development of a career track for public health professionals, establishment of regional Schools of Public Health, and institution of district level disease surveillance and epidemiology units [55].

In 1999, the South East Asia Regional Office (SEARO) of WHO conducted a conference on Public Health in South-East Asia in the twenty-first century. The main recommendations embodied in the *Calcutta Declaration on Public Health* are [56]:

> Having noted the progress in public health practice, education, training, and research in the countries of the South-East Asia Region, and having reviewed the lessons from public health-related policies and programs, we endorse the following strategies and directions for enhancing health development in the South-East Asia Region in the twenty-first Century:
>
> 1. Promote public health as a discipline and as an essential requirement for health development in the Region. In addition to addressing the challenges posed by ill-health and promoting positive health, public health should also address issues related to poverty, equity, ethics, quality, social justice, environment, community development, and globalization.
>
> 2. Recognize the leadership role of public health in formulating and implementing evidence-based healthy public policies; creating supportive environments; enhancing social responsibility by involving communities, and increasing the allocations of human and financial recourses.
>
> 3. Strengthen public health by creating career structures at national, state, provincial and district levels, and by establishing policies to mandate competent background and relevant expertise for persons responsible for the health of populations.
>
> 4. Strengthen and reform public health education, training, and research, as supported by the networking of institutions and the use of information technology, for improving human resources development.

The impact of these recommendations remains to be seen. Interestingly, the Supreme Court of India has recently banned smoking in public places as it violates the right to health of the public.

Approaches to public health training

The need for independent schools of public health has been long debated internationally. Alternative models are the integrated faculty of health sciences incorporating medicine, public health and other disciplines, and the postgraduate training of public health practitioners within medical schools. The later model is dominant in India with over one-hundred medical colleges offering postgraduate degrees for medical graduates in "preventive and social medicine" or "community medicine". These programs do not offer training in the full range of public health sciences and have not embraced the full range of health scientists needed in modern public health practice.

There is only one long standing school of public health in the western sense in South Asia, in Calcutta, established during British rule; this school has not been further developed over the last few decades. In Trivandrum, Kerala, the Achutha Menon Centre for Health Science Studies has offered a modern MPH course since 1998 but still with only a small number of students, relative to the need in India. This centre is the public health wing of the Sree Chitra Tirunal Institute for Medical Sciences and Technology. This Institute was established by an act of parliament in 1977 and is now an "institution of national importance" under the National Government Department of Science and Technology and has the status of a university.

The name of institutions is sometimes less relevant than their role and the context in which they perform (e.g., Pakistan has several "schools of public health" that train only basic levels of PHC workers). Pakistan is not a member of SEARO (it is included within WHO's Eastern Mediterranean Regional Office), and is not party to the *Calcutta Declaration*; its educational experience differs. Throughout the twentieth century, higher education in public health was largely unavailable in Pakistan, reflecting it's low priority, and most aspirants qualified abroad. However, during the 1990s, in addition to a few existing diploma programs, a national Health Services Academy was formed, several institutions launched MPH degrees, others developed specialized Masters degrees (e.g., epidemiology, health policy), and specialty certification in community medicine became available for physicians through active programs (having been on the books for decades) [57]. Community based learning is now recommended for all medical colleges [58], and community health nursing emerged as a recognized nursing specialty [59].

Professional education in public health disciplines is also developing in Sri Lanka, Bangladesh, and Nepal. For example, the Bangladesh Rural Advancement Committee (BRAC) is developing plans for a new school of public health [60]. Together with the observations from India and Pakistan, it seems that modern public health education is slowly taking hold in South Asia. Challenges remain: public sector institutions often suffer from being administered within inefficient ministerial bureaucracies, accreditation systems (where they exist) are generally immature and sometimes capricious, the tradition of rote learning must be broken in favour of problem solving [61]; the under-education of women means that the medical profession remains male dominated, while nursing is viewed unfavorably by most Muslim families [62]; standards vary widely, and sustainability of some programs is fragile. The output also is still much less than required, and many candidates still leave to study in costly but often less appropriate programs abroad, although government recruiting policies and career pathways are becoming more favorable. Modern public health training must be complemented by serious attention to professional career structures and human resource planning.

On an encouraging note, teaching field sites in several countries, for example the International Centre for Diarrhoeal Disease Research in Bangladesh, have contributed new tools, methods, technologies, and strategies, and have demonstrated how major health improvements may be achieved locally [63,64]. Participating communities have become better organized and there are significant impacts at provincial and national levels. Without the demonstration power of such initiatives (linked to community based education), there would be even greater pressure to develop health services in line with the traditional medical approach that, despite relevance to diagnosis and treatment, are unable to meet public health needs. Regardless of how organized or labeled, developing professional education options in public health is critical in all countries in the region.

Related issues of health reform

"Health care reform" in South Asia, as elsewhere, is driven more by fiscal than by health priorities. While there is a need to improve managerial efficiency, a fundamental reality is ignored: no region anywhere in the world has achieved favourable health outcomes with such low public expenditure on health, especially when this is mostly diverted to curative services. Although the concept of "investing in health" is not yet recognized by political leaders, there is some hope in a growing perception that health reform offers opportunities for devolution of power and more local governance. This opportunity could be harnessed to strengthen public health, including environmental standards, surveillance, and prevention and control of locally prevalent diseases (not just those deemed globally important).

In most South Asian countries, health, education and rural development suffer from distortions in priority setting, insufficient fiscal allocations, and poor management. For example, in India and Pakistan, governmental health expenditures comprise little more than half of one percent of all public expenditures (debt servicing and military expenditures take the lion's share); the bulk of the health budget goes to hospitals (70 percent in India, the highest in Asia) [65]. As a consequence of the minimum investment in health, private providers now dominate the sector (80 percent of health services in Pakistan), with minimal regulation [66]. This development was not guided by any policy vision. Equally lacking are explicit social development objectives to underpin the development of community participation, an essential ingredient in meaningful health reform [67].

To achieve community-based health service developments, strategies to promote participation and gender equity are required. Unfortunately, most public sector managers have little training or experience in community development models; this expertise exists mainly in nongovernmental organizations (NGOs), and must therefore be tapped if progress is to be made.

Effective public–private synergies exist. In the remote hill districts of Nepal, where infrastructure is poor, tuberculosis control (including home visits) is supported by an international NGO [68]. Disease control and supporting research is carried out in Bangladesh by the Danish Bangladesh Leprosy Mission [69]. Also in Bangladesh, BRAC (a national NGO) covers more than thirty million people for directly observed short course treatment (DOTS) for tuberculosis and operates many other important social and economic initiatives [70]. In Sri Lanka, Sarvodaya implements a community health program integrated within a rural community development network [71]. The Aga Khan Development Network is participating with 100 villages in the northern areas of Pakistan to improve water, sanitation and hygiene education, and working with government to develop PHC. In several countries family planning associations and social marketing organizations are forces for policy change and supply contraceptive programming. However, although NGOs have this potential to support public health objectives, most partnerships to date entail small scale projects with limited budgets and restrictive timeframes. Furthermore, the private sector generally is absent in public policy debates, which is a lost opportunity for dialogue. Public sector leaders talk about fostering partnerships, but to achieve action the private sector must also be part of this debate. It is equally critical that governments in South Asia accept more fully their responsibility for public health and to prioritize, plan and budget accordingly.

The intended outcomes of partnerships include extending services to meet human needs, improving management, enhancing local capacities, and reorganizing systems to become more responsive [72]. Partnership emphasizes working together, rather than the tradition of "two solitudes", which leads to suboptimal performance from either sector [73]. In the interests of its people, South Asia must get on with forming partnerships that work, and developing the norms and standards to guide the adequacy, accessibility and quality of health services.

The way forward

The road ahead will be difficult, despite an apparent increase in international agency recognition for the link between poverty and health burdens in developing countries. For example, the Global Fund to Fight AIDS, Tuberculosis and Malaria, reflects a continuing emphasis on vertical programming for a few diseases deemed to be global priorities [74]. Similarly, despite a broader scope, the Commission on Macroeconomics and Health advocates "essential interventions"; implicitly these are "selective PHC" approaches which require mostly top-down decisions with little reference to building local capacity [75]. While these reports emphasize the "disease to poverty" pathway, the alternative model (i.e., "poverty to disease") requires at least equal emphasis in local actions and is more firmly established in the literature. While The People's Health Assembly was effective in eliciting a response from the Director General of WHO [76,77], this was more concerned with the perceptions of the G8 group of countries and the role of industry in supplying products and services, than the principle of community participation that lies at the heart of PHC. Public health in South Asia must not be left to the international community to define; it is primarily the responsibility of the countries themselves to define their priorities. The global agenda should be viewed as complementary at best, and South Asian countries must build their systems more assertively in accordance with their public health needs and with their own resources.

Alleviation of South Asia's poor health status requires better priority setting by governments and increased investment to achieve universal education and improved public health performance. It demands principled leadership, responsible governance, ethical and innovative management, informed choices, and participation by people in decisions affecting their health. Above all, improving population health in this region, as elsewhere, depends on social and economic development, especially literacy and gender equity, as well as sound public health initiatives.

References

[1] Mather RJ, John TJ. Popular beliefs about smallpox and other common infectious diseases. *Tropical and Geographic Medicine* 1973; 25: 190–6.

[2] Thankappan KR. Some health implications of globalization in Kerala, India. *Bull WHO* 2001; 79: 892–3.

[3] Ahmad OB, Lopez AD, Inoue M. Decline in child mortality: a reappraisal. *Bull WHO* 2000; 78: 1175–91.

[4] Halstead SB, Walsh JA, Warren KS (eds.). *Good Health at Low Cost.* New York: Rockefeller Foundation, 1985.

[5] National Sample Survey Organization. Morbidity and treatment of ailments. NSS fifty-second round, July 1995–June 1996. Report No. 441. New Delhi: Ministry of Health, Government of India.

[6] John TJ, Samuel R, Balraj V, John R. Disease surveillance at district level: a model for developing countries. *Lancet* 1998; 352: 58–61.

[7] Population Reference Bureau, 2001 World Population Data Sheet.

[8] United Nations Development Programme, *Human Development Report 2000*. New York: Oxford University Press, 2000.

[9] United Nations. *World Population Prospects, Vol. II*. New York: Economic and Social Affairs. 1998.

[10] Omran AR. The epidemiologic transition. A theory of the epidemiology of population change. *The Milbank Memorial Fund Quarterly* 1971; **49**: 509–38.

[11] Hill K, Abou Zahr C, Wardlaw T. Estimates of maternal mortality for 1995. *Bull WHO* 2001; **79**: 182–93.

[12] Jafarey SN, Korejo R. Mothers brought dead: an inquiry into causes of delay. *Soc Sci Med* 1993; **36**: 371–2.

[13] Tinker AG. Improving women's health in Pakistan. *Health, Nutrition, and Population Series*. Washington: The World Bank, 1998.

[14] Goodburn E, Chowdhury M, Gazi R et al. Training traditional birth attendants in clean delivery does not prevent postpartum infection. *Health Policy and Planning* 2000; **15**: 394–9.

[15] The global elimination of neonatal tetanus: progress to date. *Bull WHO* 1994; **72**: 155–64.

[16] Bennet J, Ma C, Traverso H, Agha BS, Boring J. Neonatal tetanus associated with topical unmbilical ghee: covert use of cow dung. *Int J Epidemiol* 1999; **28**: 1172–5.

[17] UNICEF State of the World's Children 2001. New York: UNICEF, 2001.

[18] Murray CJL, Lopez AD. The *Global Burden of Disease*. Geneva: World Health Organization, 1996.

[19] Mathur ML, Khatri PK, Base CS. Drug resistance in tuberculosis patients in Joghpur district. *Indian J Med Sci* 2000; **54**: 55–8.

[20] Kidson C, Indaratna K. Ecology, economics and political will: the vicissitudes of malaria strategies in Asia. *Parassitologia* 1998; **40**: 39–46.

[21] Bhutta ZA. The challenge of multidrug resistant typhoid in childhood: current status and prospects for the future. *Indian Pediatr* 1999; **36**: 129–31.

[22] Khan AJ, Luby SP, Fikree F et al. Unsafe injections and the transmission of hepatitis B and C in a periurban community in Pakistan. *Bull WHO* 2000; **78**: 956–63.

[23] Sehgal S. HIV epidemic in Punjab, India: time trends over a decade. *Bull WHO* 1998; **76**: 509–13.

[24] Srikanth P, John TJ, Jeyakumari H et al. Epidemiological features of acquired immunodeficiency syndrome in southern India. *Indian J Med Res*. 1997; 105191–7.

[25] Nanan D, Kadir MM, White F. Survey and surveillance development in settings with low HIV prevalence. *Eastern Med Health J* 2000; **6**: 670–7.

[26] Hawkes S, Morison L, Foster S et al. Reproductive tract infection in women in low-income, low prevalence situation: assessment of syndromic management in Matlab, Bangladesh. *Lancet* 1999; **354**: 1776–81.

[27] Goldenberg RL, Andrews WW, Yuan AC, MacKay HT, St Louis ME. Sexually transmitted diseases and adverse outcomes of pregnancy. *Clin Perinatol* 1997; **24**: 23–41.

[28] McKeigue PM. Coronary heart disease in Indians, Pakistanis, and Bangladeshis: aetiology and possibilities for prevention. *Brit Heart J* 1992; **67**: 341–2.

[29] Stein CE, Fall CHD, Kumaran K et al. Fetal growth and coronary heart disease in south India. *Lancet* 1996; **348**: 1269–73.

[30] King H, Aubert RE, Herman WH. Global burden of diabetes, 1995–2025. *Diabetes Care*. 1998; **21**: 1414–31.

[31] White F, Rafique G. Diabetes prevalence and projections in South Asia: an emerging public health priority for the 21st century. *Selected Proc. 9th International Congress*. World Fed Pub Hlth Associations. 2–6 Sept. 2000 Beijing, China. APHA Washington, 2001, pp. 118–20.

[32] Nanan D, White F. The National Health Survey of Pakistan. Review and discussion of report findings pertaining to selected risk factors for cardio-vascular disease. *ProCOR Digest* 1999; **99**: 6–11. (http://www.procor.org/procor-community-hma/msg00006.html)

[33] White F. Developing effective and affordable models for non-communicable disease prevention and control. *Int J Epidemiol* 2001; **30**: 1494–5.

[34] Dowse GK, Gareeboo H, Alberti KJMM et al. Changes in population cholesterol concentrations and other cardiovascular risk factor levels after five years of the non-communicable disease intervention programme in Mauritius. *BMJ* 1995; **311**: 1255–9.

[35] Pan XR, Li GW, Hu YH et al. Effects of diet and exercise in preventing NIDDM in people with impaired glucose tolerance. The Da Qing IGT and diabetes study. *Diabetes Care* 1997; **20**: 537–44.

[36] Rabbani F, Raja FF. The minds of mothers: maternal mental health in an urban squatter settlement of Karachi. *J Pak Med Assoc* 2000; **50**: 306–12.

[37] Hussain R, Fikree FF, Berendes HW. The role of son preference in reproductive behaviour in Pakistan. *Bull WHO* 2000; **78**: 379–88.

[38] Sen A. *Development as Freedom*. New York: Anchor Books, 1999.

[39] Mitra S. Factors in the sociocultural environment of child labourers: a study in a small scale leather goods industry in Calcutta. *Occup Environ Med* 1994; **51**: 822–5.

[40] George AM (ed.). Lead poisoning prevention & treatment: implementing a national program in developing countries. *Proceedings of the International Conference on lead Poisoning*. 8–10 February, 1999. The George Foundation. Bangalore 1999. www.leadpoison.net.

[41] Merchant A, Husain SSM, Hosain M et al. Paan without tobacco: an independent risk factor for oral cancer. *Int J Cancer* 2000; **86**: 128–31.

[42] Ghaffar A, Hyder A, Mastoor MI, Shaikh I. Injuries in Pakistan: directions for future health policy. *Health Policy and Planning* 1999; **14**: 11–17.

[43] Primary Health Care. A joint report by the Director General of the World Health Organization and the Executive Director of the United Nations Children's Fund. New York: World Health Organization, 1978.

[44] Walsh JA, Warren KS. Selective primary health care: an interim strategy for disease control in developing countries. *NEJM* 1979; **301**: 967–74.

[45] Walsh J, Warren KS (eds.). *Strategies for Primary Health Care. Technologies appropriate for the control of disease in the Developing World.* Chicago: University of Chicago Press, 1986.

[46] World Health Organization. World Health Report, 2000. Geneva: World Health Organization, 2000.

[47] Hopkins DR, Azam M, Ruiz-Tiben E, Kappus KD. Eradication of dracunculiasis from Pakistan. *Lancet* 1995; **346**: 621–4.

[48] World Health Organization. Dracunculiasis. Weekly Epidemiological Record 2001. http://www.who.int/ctd/dracun.

[49] Karmarker MG, Pandav CS. Interpretation of indicators of iodine deficiency disorders: recent experiences. *Natl Med J India* 1999; **12**: 113–17.

[50] Anderson RM, May RM. Age related changes in the rate of disease transmission: implications for the design of vaccination programs. *J Hyg (Lond)* 1985; **94**: 365–436.

[51] People's Charter for Health. PHA Secretariat, Gonoshasthaya Kendra, Savar, Dhaka, 1344, Bangladesh. http://www.pha2000.org.

[52] Cash RA, Narasimhan V. Impediments to global surveillance of infectious diseases: consequences of open reporting in a global economy. *Bull WHO* 2000; **78**: 1358–67.

[53] Editorial, The Plague Within. The Hindu, 21 February, 2002.

[54] Technical Advisory Committee on Plague. Report of the Expert Committee on Plague, August 1995. Ministry of Health and Family Welfare, New Delhi: Government of India.

[55] Expert Committee on Public Health System. Report of the Expert Committee on Public Health System, May 1996. Ministry of Health and Family Welfare, New Delhi: Government of India.

[56] Anon. Calcutta Declaration on Public Health. *J Health Pop Dev Countries* 2000; **3**: 5.

[57] White F. Community Medicine—a specialty whose time has come. *J Coll Phys Surg Pakistan* 2001; **11**: 733–5.

[58] Bryant JH, Marsh D, Khan K et al. A developing country's university oriented toward strengthening health systems: challenges and results. *AJPH* 1993; **83**: 1537–43.

[59] Harner R, Burns J, Marshall P, Karmarliani R. Community based nursing in Pakistan. *J Contin Educ Nurs* 1994; **25**: 130–2.

[60] Bryant J, Cash R. Feasibility study on the development of a School of Public Health at BRAC University, Dhaka, Bangladesh—14 January to 3 February 2002. Unpublished document.

[61] Rahbar MH, Vellani C, Sajan F et al. Predictability of medical students' performances at the Aga Khan University from admission test scores, interview ratings and systems of education. *Medical Education* 2001; **35**: 374–80.

[62] Haq MB. Lady health visitors: public health nursing education in Pakistan. *J Cult Divers* 1994; **1**: 36–40.

[63] Rabbani F. A view of the city's health from The Aga Khan University, Karachi, Pakistan. *Urban Health and Development Bulletin. Medical Research Council, South Africa* 1999; **2**: 99–111.

[64] ICDDR,B: Centre for Health and Population Research. 2002 http://www.icddrb.org.

[65] Griffin CC. Health care in Asia: A comparative study of cost and financing. Washington: World Bank Regional and Sectoral Studies, 1992.

[66] National Health Survey of Pakistan. Pakistan Medical Research Council. Islamabad, 1998.

[67] Asian Development Bank. Health sector reform in Asia and the Pacific: options for developing countries. Manila, 1999.

[68] White AJ, Robinson-White CM, Luitel H. A report on home visiting practices conducted in remote districts of Nepal in an NGO-run tuberculosis control program. *Int J Tuberc Lung Dis* 1999; **3**: 534–6.

[69] Croft RP. Active surveillance in leprosy: how useful is it? *Lepr Rev* 1996; **67**: 135–40.

[70] Islam A, Nakamura Y, Wonkhomthong S-A, Chowdhury SA, Ishikawa N. Involvement of community health workers in tuberculosis control in Bangladesh. *Jpn J Trop Med Hyg* 1999; **27**: 167–73.

[71] Sarvodaya Shramadana Movement. www.sarvodaya.org.

[72] Working with private sector providers for better health care: an introductory guide. Options Consultancy Services Ltd. & London School of Hygiene and Tropical Medicine. London, 2001.

[73] Widdus R. Public-private partnerships for health: their main targets, their diversity, and their future directions. *Bull WHO* 2001; **79**: 713–20.

[74] Brundtland GH, Piot P. The Global Fund to fight AIDS, Tuberculosis and Malaria, Pre-Board Meeting. Office of the Director General. World Health Organization, 27 January 2002. www.who.int/director-general/spe...2/english/20020127_globalfundboard.html.

[75] Report of the Commission on Macroeconomics and Health. *Macroeconomics and Health: Investing in Health for Development*. Geneva: World Health Organization, 2001. www.cmhealth.org.

[76] Chowdhury Z. The People's Health Assembly. *BMJ* 2000; **321**: 1361–2.

[77] Brundtland GH. The People's Health Assembly. *BMJ* 2001; **323**: 109.

Chapter 11

Public health in Australia and New Zealand

Peter Davis and Vivian Lin

Introduction

Public health in Australia and New Zealand reflects a special set of historical and geographical circumstances expressed by some of the most favorable health outcomes in the world. The pattern reached its height in the 1950s and 1960s with cultural and social protection, political and economic stability, and relative insulation. Since then these conditions have been largely dissipated, both by reforming governments [1] and by the pressures of globalization and regional transformation. This chapter reviews the unique historical experience of public health in these two countries, evaluates their more recent achievements, and assesses their likely prospects in rapidly changing regional and global circumstances.

Societal context

Australia and New Zealand represent the furthest and final reach of the British colonial venture. Despite this common historical heritage, there are important differences between the two countries. These are to be seen in: political system—Australia is federal, New Zealand unitary; in levels of migration—high and varied for Australia, New Zealand traditionally low and controlled; in size, standard of living, economic and demographic growth—all more developed in Australia; and in focus of regional engagement—Australia towards Asia, New Zealand to the South Pacific. In most important respects, however, the two countries have much in common.

Beyond these distinctive historical and societal features, both countries share many features relevant to public health with the rest of the developed world. For example, with affluence and the demographic transition have come ageing of their populations. Economic deregulation has been associated with the decline of protected industries and growing social inequality. Changes in the role of women and in home and family life have accompanied industrial restructuring and shifts in patterns and levels of workforce participation. Overlaying these fundamental demographic, economic and social changes are important ideological movements—individual rights, women, labour, indigenous peoples, the environment—and major shifts in perceptions of health and the role of the State. These cultural and ideological movements have much in common with the recent historical experience of other economically developed societies.

Health and policy context

Both Australia and New Zealand are at a stage of the epidemiological transition characteristic of other economically advanced societies. Both countries have well developed welfare states and elaborate administrative and governance structures. Policy is also heavily influenced, and delivered, by a range of nongovernmental bodies in the health field. Finally, both countries have undergone nearly a quarter of a century of structural reform and change in the health field, much of it oscillating between competing political tendencies and ideological perspectives [2].

Epidemiological transition

Australia and New Zealand follow the pattern of societies that advanced through the late stages of the epidemiological transition. Both have birth rates below replacement levels, substantial populations in the retirement years, display a pattern of ill-health, including mental health problems, that has moved well beyond the communicable diseases, with relatively low levels of mortality [3], and both enjoy superior life expectancy and rapidly advancing health expectancy [4] (Table 11.1).

A feature of both societies is subpopulations which vary in their progress through the health transition and which differ markedly in health experience. Australian Aborigines still have high birth and death rates and high rates of communicable disease. New Zealand Maori have only recently passed through the transition, and some Pacific groups are still showing high birth rates. Furthermore, the favorable statistics on life and health expectancy (Table 11.1) are those of the majority populations of European origin, particularly those in affluent circumstances. The indigenous population groups, together with other disadvantaged socioeconomic and ethnic groups, fare much more poorly in health outcomes [8,9].

Table 11.1 Demographic indicators in New Zealand and Australia

Demographic indicators	New Zealand[1] [5]	Australia[2] [6]
Total population	3.8 million	18.9 million
Percentage population over sixty-five	11.6%	12.2%
Total fertility rate	1.9	1.7
Infant mortality rate (deaths per 1000 live births)	5.6	5.0
Life expectancy at birth—males	75.2	75.9
Life expectancy at birth—females	80.4	81.5
Disability-adjusted life expectancy [7]	69.2	73.2

[1] Data for 1998, except for disability-adjusted life expectancy (1999).
[2] Data for 1999, except life expectancy statistics (1998).

Table 11.2 Economic indicators, New Zealand and Australia

Economic indicators	New Zealand[1] [5]	Australia[2] [6]
Percentage of GPD on health	8.2	8.5
Percentage of health expenditure private	22.5	28.8
Percentage of health budget allocation on public health	1.7	1.8–2.0

[1] Data for 1999.
[2] Data for 2000, except public health (1999) [10].

Welfare state tradition

Australia and New Zealand follow the tradition of the other English-speaking democracies in taxation and welfare state provision. While clearly committed to a comprehensive system of social protection and State involvement in health and education and a range of other fields, the levels of taxation and public funding in these countries do not match those of many European countries. The level of private funding for health care in Australia and New Zealand is substantial, but close to the OECD average. Overall funding as a percentage of GDP also registers close to where one might expect these countries to be, given their relative position of national wealth (Table 11.2).

Administrative and governance structures

While Australia and New Zealand follow the "Westminster" tradition of parliamentary government, and share a similar party political structure, they diverge on key institutional features. New Zealand has a unitary system, a single-chamber parliament, and election is by proportional representation. There is also a historical treaty relationship with Maori, with its own associated strand of public health development (see Box 11.1). Australia, by contrast, is a federation with a considerable dilution of central government power through the principle of subsidiarity (powers are exercised by the states, or as close as possible to the community, unless stipulated otherwise by the constitution). The Australian parliament has two chambers and is elected by a process that is closer to the traditional constituency system (at least for the lower house). There is no formal

Box 11.1   Maori health initiatives

New Zealand's earliest hospitals dated from the 1840s. These were intended primarily for use by the indigenous people, but the rapidly increasing white settler population soon displaced Maori patients in most localities. From the 1850s central government subsidised general practitioners to treat Maori. From the 1890s until the late 1930s, when universal medical benefits were introduced under the First Labour Government, approximately one-sixth of all GPs were engaged in this scheme. In 1920 the Department established a separate Division of Maori Hygiene, headed by a Maori doctor. This was disbanded in 1930 when responsibility for Maori health was returned to the medical officers of health [11].

Disparities between Maori and nonMaori health increasingly exercised the minds of politicians and policymakers from the 1930s. The catalyst was the revelation that Maori had a far higher incidence and mortality for key indicators such as infant mortality and tuberculosis. Until the 1980s, acceptance of western medicine, together with improved economic and housing conditions, was seen as the solution to Maori health problems. A growing commitment to Maori self-determination, however, saw the introduction of "by Maori for Maori" health services during the 1990s. There was also a revival of traditional healing, whose practitioners, the tohunga, had been outlawed in 1907. By the mid-1990s there were about 200 traditional healing clinics operating in New Zealand.

recognition of indigenous rights in the Australian constitutional system and Aboriginal Australians did not gain the right to vote until 1968.

Despite the difference in constitutional character, both countries have experienced similar challenges and trajectories in the delivery of health services, including public health. Thus, initially, public health functions were jealously defended at the local level, with central government relegated to a broad regulatory role. However, issues of funding and the threat of epidemics moved such responsibilities "upwards" so that, by 1900 in New Zealand [12] and by 1901 in Victoria, Australia, public health legislation building on the late-nineteenth century Public Health Acts in England was passed establishing governmental agencies with responsibilities in the area. In both countries central government responsibilities in health care only crystallized and grew rapidly in the second half of the twentieth century. Local government retained key powers in environmental health and regulation.

A turbulent period

The period since the early 1970s has been one of partisanship, ideological debate and almost constant health system restructuring. Issues of public health have been a major theme and, to an important extent, a litmus test of wider philosophical trends. The 1970s saw a renewed commitment from left-of-centre governments in both countries to public investment in health, most strikingly with Medibank in Australia. The debate over the role of the State re-ignited in the late-1980s with the return of similar governments, while the 1990s saw a trend towards health restructuring stimulated by neo-liberal concepts [13]. This also coincided with a weakening of public health commitments at the political and bureaucratic level, with savage budget cuts across the health system in Australian states.

The debates of the 1970s resulted in greater campaigning and activism in public health, fuelled by broader social and ideological changes [14]. This was a challenge to the "old public health" and brought in an active health promotion agenda. These gains were consolidated with a refreshing of national institutions in the 1980s. This was particularly evident in Australia [15]. Both countries initiated goals and targets, major screening programmes, and significant initiatives on HIV/AIDS and tobacco control. These advances were slowed, but not entirely reversed, in an environment in the 1990s that was ideologically and politically more hostile to public health. Indeed, the Australian National Public Health Partnership was an initiative from public health officials to strengthen the system and to respond to the challenges from new public sector management [16].

Public health infrastructure

In its origins, public health emerged in Australia and New Zealand strongly influenced by the model of Britain. This early legal and legislative framework has had an enduring influence, but more important since has been the particular logistical and health challenges of both countries. As ever, the resourcing and administrative arrangements for the public health function have been matters of controversy. Nevertheless, there are some notable achievements in the information base for public health decision-making, in workforce development, and in research and development activities. These areas are all fluid and under constant negotiation, but, despite setbacks and a lack of consistent and long-term strategic guidance and development, they suggest there is a considerable vigour and creativity underpinning public health in Australia and New Zealand.

Legal framework

The origins of the legal framework for the public health function in both countries lie in the great legislative initiatives of late-nineteenth century Victorian Britain. While the early settlers assumed that they were escaping the worst excesses of industrial Europe, many of the conditions of urban squalor were replicated in the Antipodes. These circumstances, together with concerns about the potential for the spread of epidemic disease associated with large-scale migration, prompted the early efforts to define the core public health function, establish the associated administrative structures, and secure the necessary funding. The 1918 influenza epidemic added urgency and impetus to the evolution of a public health administration. The special requirements of disadvantaged indigenous peoples and of providing coverage over large, sparsely populated areas, gave a distinct character to public health responsibilities and structures.

The role of the Medical Officer of Health was central to the early public health framework, and remains important to this day. As defined in the early legislation, the Medical Officer of Health had important statutory responsibilities for the control of communicable disease—particularly epidemics and outbreaks—and around this core function was established the broader range of health protection duties, generally also of a regulatory and enforcement character. To the early responsibilities in infectious disease control were added food safety and hygiene, venereal disease, aspects of living and environmental conditions (generally handled by local rather than central government), general monitoring and surveillance activities, and screening (for example, tuberculosis).

The agenda of the "new public health"—a mixture of non-communicable and novel communicable disease challenges—extended the legal and enforcement mandate of public health (for example, tobacco control and alcohol licensing). But it also complemented this traditional function with the educational and empowerment strategies of health promotion. The Ottawa Charter provided a complementary vision and regulatory strategy. Further to this, concerns with privacy, confidentiality and non-discrimination—as in the case of HIV/AIDS—elaborated and complicated the once more straightforward legal basis for the public health function. Monitoring and surveillance no longer went uncontested. More "positive" duties have also been added. The ability to conduct health impact assessment of public policy proposals in Tasmania, to develop municipal public health plans in Victoria and Queensland, and to fund health promotion activities through tobacco tax hypothecation (Box 11.2), have been some recent Australian achievements. Novel legal and ethical issues are also emerging with the new genetics. Thus in the case of GMOs, the appropriate balance between the precautionary principle—fundamental to the public health ethos—and the growth and development oriented agendas of key economic and scientific interests has been in contention.

Box 11.2   Health promotion foundations

In 1987, the Victorian Parliament passed the Tobacco Act—the first act of its kind internationally—setting aside a portion of the tax on tobacco sales for health promotion activities [17]. The passage of the legislation was achieved with active lobbying by a broad coalition, led by the Anti-Cancer Council of Victoria, and underpinned by substantial health and economic research and public opinion surveys. The Act banned advertising of tobacco products at public events (with limited exemptions such as the Grand Prix), and, as a trade-off, the arts and sports sponsorship was "bought out" by the Victorian Health Promotion Foundation. In doing so, the Foundation required art and sporting organizations to enter into partnerships with health sector organizations to promote health messages. In addition, the Foundation funded community-based health promotion programmes and public health research.

Western Australia, South Australia, and the Australian Capital Territory have also passed similar legislation and established equivalent bodies. In 1996, the tobacco industry was successful in having the Federal High Court declare the state taxation arrangements to be unconstitutional. As a consequence, the tax is now collected by the Commonwealth and transferred to the state treasuries, who then provide the foundations with their budgets.

Administrative structures

The fortunes of public health have always been closely associated with the activities of the State. The legal and regulatory frameworks exemplify that relationship. However, with these powers and responsibilities have come potentially complicated administrative arrangements. In both Australia and New Zealand there has been a tension between centralism and localism. With the abolition of the provinces in New Zealand in 1867, public health became a central government function. But the exact deployment of public health services has oscillated between central government—the Department and then Ministry of Health—and various local and regional agencies as the New Zealand system has undergone a series of reorganizations. Added to this is the role of local government in delivering environmental and resource management services.

With its unitary and unicameral political system, there has never been any doubt about the national and uniform application of public health legislation in New Zealand. Certainly, the reforms of the 1990s seemed set to erect, for a country of fewer than four million, a relatively complicated structure of advisory, purchasing and delivery agencies running in parallel to personal health services, but the mandate was a unitary and national one [18]. In the case of Australia, however, jurisdiction at the level of the states has led not only to conflict with the Commonwealth but also to difficulties in ensuring national uniformity. For example, a nationally consistent list of notifiable diseases was achieved only in 2000.

Financing and resource allocation

Just as the rise of public health has historically been associated with the growing role of the State in social stewardship, so the financial viability of the sector has been closely tied to the fortunes of government. In the early stages of development public health was reliant on the uncertain and variable support of local government. It was this inconstancy in financial support, and the lack of adherence to fundamental public health precautions—particularly in times of epidemic threat—that forced central government in New Zealand, and state and federal authorities in Australia, to take on both financial and administrative responsibility for public health. To the basic role of disease control and related enforcement functions have been added other activities in the areas of prevention, such as maternal and child health services, school dental services, and services for indigenous peoples. Other related areas of expenditures that are sometimes considered to be in the broad realm of public health touch upon primary care, where immunization and other preventive activities receive special funding and administrative support.

In Australia and New Zealand the proportion of "health vote" directed to core public health functions has rarely risen above two percent (see Table 11.2). This figure is in line with that for other developed countries. This funding has come exclusively out of taxation. In addition, governments have supplemented tax-based support with funding from ad hoc sources (see Box 11.2). For example, state governments in Australia have experimented with tobacco tax-hypothecated health promotion foundations. While this additional funding for health promotion was welcomed, this also allowed health authorities to "cost shift" and move out of directly funding these activities in some instances. For instance, as part of budget cuts in 1991, Health Department Victoria shed its entire health promotion unit of about 90 staff, and the recurrent cost of a range of public health programmes was passed on to the Victorian Health Promotion Foundation during the 1993 budget cuts.

In New Zealand the reforms of 1990s affected the stability, mix and rationale of funding for public health. The incorporation of central government regional public health services into the Area Health Boards of the late 1980s seemed to herald a historic realignment in which the public health agenda would take its rightful place alongside that of the personal health services in a set of fully regionalised health authorities. Instead, this period into the early 1990s was one of retrenchment. Core public health functions remained, but resources and personnel ebbed away with the pressure from clinical services and the unravelling of the infrastructure of public health nursing [19]. The funding of public health remained in reduced circumstances through the 1990s, despite an attempt to establish an independent advisory authority—the Public Health Commission (Box 11.3)—and despite the re-emergence (and de-integration) of regional public health services [18]. Supplementary funding for public health only came in Maori health (sometimes controversially, as in the case of the special contributions to a campaign on Hepatitis B).

Controversies of the kind associated with the implementation of new programmes, for example major screening initiatives [21], have raised issues about the proper economic evaluation of public health when assessed alongside the demands for resources in personal health. With increasing concern from governments about "value for money", the desirability of greater economic analyses (such as cost-effectiveness analysis) has been expressed. These tools have not been used extensively, in part because of the paucity of appropriate data, and in part because most decision-making is based around changes at the margins. Programme-based Marginal Analysis (PBMA) has been one tool used, particularly in New South Wales and South Australia, because it better approximates

Box 11.3   The public health commission

In 1993 the New Zealand government established the Public Health Commission as part of sweeping health reforms. The Commission had three functions: intelligence, policy, and contracting. The integration of these functions allowed the Public Health Commission to undertake needs assessment as a basis for evidence-based policy and programmes that could then be directly contracted with service providers.

In just over two years, the Commission produced two annual state of the nation health reports, seven public health intelligence reports, twenty-four policy papers, twenty-one sets of guidelines, twenty fact sheets, a wholesale revision of national health education materials, and established new models for public health service funding. The Commission's success resulted from its singularity of purpose and to some extent a degree of independence from the day-to-day demands of core government departments.

Despite these successes, the Public Health Commission was disbanded in 1995 with its functions reintegrated into the Ministry of Health and regional health authorities. The demise of the Commission resulted from a combination of opposing industry (tobacco and alcohol) pressure, bureaucratic rivalry and a ministerial preference for closer proximity of the public health function [20].

administrative decision-making [22]. The New Zealand Ministry has developed the use of data from Burden of Disease analyses and information on inequality to prioritise public health strategies [23]. The government pharmaceutical purchasing agency has applied cost-utility analyses to drug subsidy decisions, just as its Australian counterpart applies a stringent cost-effectiveness analysis. However, the application of systematic economic analyses of this kind remains limited, while public health authorities struggle with new approaches for financing and resource allocation (Box 11.4).

Investment in intellectual and human capital

One of the key issues in the infrastructure for public health relates to the investment in what one might call the intellectual and human capital required

Box 11.4 Aboriginal health expenditure

During the mid-1990s, conservative political forces at the federal level in Australia loudly claimed that far too much health funding was being spent on Aboriginal health, with very little returns. Deeble [24] undertook the first study of health expenditure for Aboriginal Australians. Although the study showed that on a per capita basis, the expenditure was marginally higher for Aboriginal Australians, once the need was taken into account, there was a case for increased expenditure. In fact, a breakdown of the expenditure by level of government showed that the Commonwealth outlays—through Medicare benefits and pharmaceutical benefits—was well below the average Australian. This research has formed the basis for major health system reform in the Northern Territory, where Aboriginal Australians account for about 25 percent of the population.

for the performance of core public health functions. These relate to information base, research and development (R&D), and workforce development.

Australia and New Zealand have progressively enhanced their national collections of health data. For example, since the 1970s there has been a gradual but continuous process of aligning the collection of hospital morbidity data to national definitions and minimum data sets. By contrast, it has been more difficult to forge population health data into a coherent system, and reliance is still placed on a range of mechanisms. These include notification (historically important in communicable disease control), registries (cancer being the best developed but still not adequate in New Zealand), and official ad hoc and regular surveys (at both federal and state level in Australia). In addition, surveys have been funded by such non-government organisations as the National Heart Foundation, and national public health strategies—like HIV, drugs, tobacco—have invested in their own surveys. This patchwork of data represents a significant commitment to having an information base for action. Yet, the potential of such data for policy and programme development and evaluation is unfulfilled, and there are still major gaps, such as psychosocial factors, social and environmental determinants of health, public health activities (outputs and expenditures), and trend data on major risk factors [25].

For both countries the issue of establishing a sustainable and adequately funded framework for R&D in public health has been long-standing. For example, the Medical Research Council in New Zealand was established in 1937 with early initiatives in preventive medicine [11]. Yet biomedical research soon overwhelmingly dominated the Council's funding priorities. In 1990 the Council was renamed the Health Research Council and a statutorily recognised public health committee established. This was modelled to an extent on an equivalent committee within the Australian counterpart, the National Health and Medical Research Council (NHMRC), which was initially set up in 1934. Under different political circumstances in the mid-1990s, however, the NHMRC took the decision to abolish a distinct public health identity. In a subsequent review of health and medical research [26], the categories of research were re-defined—away from "biomedical vs. clinical vs. public health," towards "basic vs. priority-driven". In Australia and New Zealand public health R&D remains somewhat parlous and under-resourced. Issues associated with the funding of research on the health needs of indigenous peoples and on health services further complicate the picture for public health R&D, providing both an opportunity for enhancing the public health brief and also a potential threat of spreading its meagre resources too thinly.

Public health workforce development has been a strong and continuing theme in both Australia and New Zealand. A crucial development was the emergence of post-graduate programmes in public health drawing on students well outside traditional spheres. In Australia this expansion occurred in the late 1980s within faculties of medicine, with a strong orientation towards epidemiology and public health research. This was followed by developments in non-medical institutions—health science faculties—with a strong orientation to health promotion and a foundation in the social sciences. In addition, some health authorities (New South Wales and Victoria) opted in the 1990s for stronger practice-based training programmes. This blossoming of multiple approaches and programmes has accompanied debates about the nature of the public health workforce—whether it is a speciality, a credentialled profession, a dimension of the job of other workers, or just a set of competencies that can be deployed in many (particularly inter-sectoral) tasks.

Public health strategies

Public health activities in Australia and New Zealand have shown a vigour and creativity that reflects an ability to work outside the "bureaucratic square" with groups in touch with community concerns, and to integrate these associations into sustained, strategically focussed, officially sanctioned, and funded campaigns [27]. In both countries the three most commonly recognised achievements in the past two decades are HIV prevention and control, tobacco control, and reduction in motor vehicle crashes. A review of the Australian experience with these campaigns identified three factors critical to success in each case: strategic policy direction, technical capacity, and the availability of supportive structures [28]. In both Australia and New Zealand the HIV/AIDS epidemic has largely been contained, smoking rates have fallen dramatically (although there are still concerns about young people), as have road deaths. In each case the formula for success involved some combination of community engagement and mobilisation, well-funded and targeted research, strategic regulatory change, and a climate of political support.

For all these successes, however, there remain areas of uncertainty in establishing and following through on key priorities. From the 1980s authorities in both countries sought to establish strategic priorities for action. In the Australian case this started with the report of the Better Health Commission [29], continued through the subsequent identification of official goals and targets [30], and culminated in the late-1990s with an attempt to declare a number of national health priorities and to link these targets through to monitored indicators. New Zealand went through much the same cycle, with a strong performance orientation in the health reforms of the 1990s [31], and highly elaborate health [32] and disability [33] strategies currently.

While entirely laudable as an attempt to introduce a more rational and systematic process into priority-setting and monitoring for public health, there is a degree of ambivalence about the experience. Thus many interest groups and lobbies have sought to influence the process. In the Australian instance, for example, by the end of the 1990s there were over thirty national public health strategies, including official national health priorities (CVD, cancer, injury, mental health, diabetes, and asthma) frequently competing for scarce resources rather than forging alliances for common action. In some instances politically effective lobbies have forced themselves up the list of priorities (such as the rural sector in Australia). Furthermore, it is not always clear that this engagement with the mainstream of the health system has resulted in anything more than a co-option of the health improvement agenda rather than significant gains for public health. For the moment, the policy emphasis in Australia is on clustering conditions and risk factors, such as through the development of a chronic disease prevention strategy [34], as a way of bringing resources, expertise, and interest groups into more effective working arrangements.

Primary care is one area in particular where this ambivalence about engagement with personal health services has come to the fore. In both Australia and New Zealand governments have identified a role for general practitioners in delivering disease prevention and, to a more limited extent, health promotion services [35]. This has resulted from a combination of both a desire to fund primary care more substantially and a philosophical commitment to advance a more population orientation in the organisation and funding of general practice. Also, in practical terms, governments were seeking ways to deliver on immunization targets and to enhance screening and other programmes in a growing number of areas (now including smoking, nutrition and physical activity in Australia). The public health community has been divided over these initiatives. In debates at professional forums, some have applauded the expanded efforts and resources for primary care, while others have been alarmed that GPs are being well supported to undertake activities for which they are neither trained nor well-placed to do, and in so doing potentially diverting resources out of public health.

Finally, there are areas where the public health agenda remains undeveloped. For example, there has been a tendency even in the area of communicable disease for funding to be "crisis-dependent". Thus in 1988, a large outbreak of legionnaire's disease in Wollongong led to the investment of resources into area-based public health units all across NSW. The 1997 series of food-borne disease outbreaks in Victoria led to the consolidation of whole-of-government responsibility for food safety within the health portfolio. In other areas, the public health response lags far behind the requirement. Thus, public health interventions for mental illness have been almost completely absent, with a national strategy and action plan for Australia developed only in the late 1990s and with a focus on early intervention of mental illness rather than mental health promotion [36]. Despite the development of environmental protection authorities and the rise of the environmental movement, environmental health (as a field of public health practice and as a public health concern) has largely disappeared from the public agenda and public consciousness, until recent efforts in establishing a National Environmental Health Council in Australia [37]. Hepatitis C also fails to receive public support, despite its potential to affect a large portion of the population, as does the problem of illicit drugs. Multicultural health promotion, despite the population mix, has also received little to no political and bureaucratic support, other than language services [38]. For a range of reasons—part technical, part political and ideological—the response in these areas remains reactive, rather than one pursuing a preventive strategy.

Conclusion

Public health in Australia and New Zealand presents a "mixed" picture [39]. As expected for economically developed economies, they have favourable health profiles. Yet, significant, and possibly growing, inequalities and disadvantages are in evidence, particularly among the indigenous peoples. Both countries have established public health systems with a clearly acknowledged mandate, strategic direction, and the requisite and full range of technical resources. Yet, funding, professional identity, and ideological rationale, remain contested and, at times, uncertain. There is considerable evidence of vigor, creativity and engagement with the concerns of the community, but public health is also bureaucratically constrained and sometimes at odds with powerful constituencies.

There are also a number of areas where public health needs to work outside established boundaries. Health inequalities, the health of indigenous peoples—most strikingly the Aborigines—the concerns of refugees and migrants, and mental health promotion [40], all work at the margins of traditional categories of public health analysis and action. There are also challenges of a more global nature—climate change, genetically modified organisms, emerging diseases, and the opportunities and dilemmas of the new health information technology, including e-health. Finally, the public health community has to consider its mandate. The "new public health" had provided one source of regeneration and redefinition, but it has also created persistent divisions within the profession. There still remain lines of ambivalence, between technical and advocacy models, between enforcement and empowerment strategies, between professional and lay concepts of public health, and between State-sponsored and community-inspired agendas for action. Above all, the dynamic global environment and the growing density of regional relations supply a new set of challenges for a model of public health that, to date, has been closely tethered to the administrative and financial structures of the modern nation State.

Despite these challenges and uncertainties, public health policy has evolved from a history of medical dominance to an accommodation of interest group pluralism, while public health practice has similarly shifted from a rather singular professional approach to one acknowledging multiple perspectives. There are some signs that a next stage may well be one of more integrative practice and a greater emphasis on investment for health, but much will depend on the cohesion of the profession.

Acknowledgements

Our thanks to Todd Krieble and Derek Dow for preparing the boxes on the Public Health Commission and Maori health initiatives, respectively. We

thank Cheryl Brunton, Frank Castles, Derek Dow, Stephen Duckett, and
Judith Healy for comments.

References

[1] Castles F, Gerritsen R, Vowles J. *The Great Experiment. Labour Parties and
Public Policy Transformation in Australia and New Zealand.* Auckland:
Auckland University Press, 1996.

[2] Bloom A (ed.). *Health Reform in Australia and New Zealand.* Melbourne:
Oxford University Press, 2000.

[3] Woodward A, Mathers C, Tobias M. Migrants, money and margarine:
possible explanations for Australia–New Zealand mortality differences. In:
R Eckersly, J Dixon, R Douglas (eds.). *The Social Origins of Health and
Well-being.* Cambridge: Cambridge University Press; 2001, pp. 114–28.

[4] Davis P, Mathers C, Graham P. Health expectancy in Australia and
New Zealand. In: JM Robine, C Jagger, C Mathers, E Crimmins, R Suzman,
REVES (eds.). *Determining Health Expectancies.* Chichester: John Wiley, 2002
(in press).

[5] French S, Old A, Healy J. "New Zealand". *Health Care Systems in Transition*
2001; 3: 1–128. European Observatory on Health Care Systems, Copenhagen.

[6] Hilless M, Healy J. "Australia" *Health Care Systems in Transition* 2001; 3: 1–98.
European Observatory on Health Care Systems, Copenhagen.

[7] Mathers CD, Sadana R, Salomon JA, Murray CJK, Lopez, AD. Healthy life
expectancy in 191 countries, 1999. *Lancet* 2001; **357**: 1685–91.

[8] Howden-Chapman P, Tobias, M. (eds.) *Social Inequalities in Health: New
Zealand 1999.* Wellington: Ministry of Health, 2000.

[9] Glover J, Harris K, Tennant S. *A Social Health Atlas of Australia.* Adelaide:
Public Health Information Development Unit, University of Adelaide, 1999.

[10] Australian Institute of Health and Welfare (AIHW). *National Public Health
Expenditure 1998–99.* Canberra: AIHW, 2001.

[11] Dow DA. *Maori Health and Government Policy 1840–1940.* Wellington:
Victoria University Press, 1999.

[12] Dow DA. *Safeguarding the Public Health. A History of the New Zealand
Department of Health.* Wellington: Victoria University Press, 1995.

[13] Ashton, T. The health reforms: to market and back? In: J Boston, P Dalziel,
S St. John (eds.), *Redesigning the Welfare State: Problems, Policies, Prospects.*
Auckland: Oxford University Press, 1999. pp. 134–53.

[14] Baum F. *The New Public Health: An Australian Perspective.* Melbourne:
Oxford University Press, 1999.

[15] Lin V, King C. Intergovernmental reforms in public health. In: A Bloom (ed.),
Health Reform in Australia and New Zealand. Melbourne: Oxford University
Press, 2000. pp. 251–63.

[16] Adams T, Lin V. Partnership in public health. *World Health Forum* 1998; **19**: 246–52.

[17] Galbally R. Placing prevention at the centre of health sector reform. In: A Bloom (ed.), *Health Reform in Australia and New Zealand*. Melbourne: Oxford University Press, 2000, pp. 264–76.

[18] Barnett P, Malcolm LA. To integrate or deintegrate? Fitting public health into New Zealand's reforming health system. *Euro J Pub Hlth* 1998; **8**: 79–86.

[19] Armstrong A, Bandaranayake D. *Public Health in New Zealand. Recent Changes and Future Prospects*. No. 1, Public Health Monograph Series. Wellington: Department of Public Health, Wellington School of Medicine, University of Otago, 1995.

[20] Krieble TA. *The Rise and Fall of a Crown Entity: A Case Study of the Public Health Commission*. Wellington: Victoria University of Wellington, 1996.

[21] Ministry of Health. *Investigation into Cervical Screening in the Tairawhiti Region, Health Funding Authority: Final Report*. Wellington: Ministry of Health, 2001.

[22] Deeble J. *Resource Allocation in Public Health: An Economic Approach*. Melbourne: National Public Health Partnership, 1999.

[23] Ministry of Health. *Evidence-Based Health Objectives for the New Zealand Health Strategy*. Public Health Intelligence Occasional Bulletin Number 2. Wellington: Ministry of Health, 2001.

[24] Deeble J. *Expenditures on Health Services for Aboriginal and Torres Strait Islander people*. Canberra: Commonwealth Department of Health and Family Services and Australian Institute of Health and Welfare, 1998.

[25] National Public Health Partnership. *National Public Health Information Development Plan*. Melbourne: National Public Health Partnership, 1999.

[26] Health and Medical Research Strategic Review Committee. *The Virtuous Cycle. Working Together for Health and Medical Research*. Canberra: Department of Health and Aged Care, 1999.

[27] National Public Health Partnership. *Key Achievements in Public Health*. Melbourne: National Public Health Partnership, 1998.

[28] National Health and Medical Research Council. *Health Australia Review*. Canberra: Health Advancement Standing Committee, 1997.

[29] Commonwealth Department of Health. *Report of the Better Health Commission*. Canberra: Australian Government Printers, 1985.

[30] Australian Health Ministers Advisory Council. *Health for All Australians: Report of the Health Goals and Targets Committee*. Canberra: Australian Government Printers, 1988.

[31] Ministry of Health. *Progress on Health Outcomes Targets. Te Haere Whamua ki nga Whainga hua mo te hauora*. Wellington: Ministry of Health, 1996.

[32] Ministry of Health. *The New Zealand Health Strategy*. Wellington: Ministry of Health, 2000.

[33] Ministry of Health. *The New Zealand Disability Strategy: Making a World of Difference*. Wellington: Ministry of Health, 2001.

[34] National Public Health Partnership. *Strategic Framework for Chronic Disease Prevention*. Melbourne: National Public Health Partnership, 2001.

[35] General Practice/Population Health Joint Action Group. *Consultation Paper: General Practice and Population Health*. Canberra: Department of Health and Aged Care, 2001.

[36] Australian Health Ministers Advisory Council. *National Mental Health Promotion and Prevention Action Plan*. Canberra: Commonwealth Department of Health and Aged Care, 1999.

[37] National Public Health Partnership, EnHealth Council, and Commonwealth Department of Health and Aged Care. *National Environmental Health Strategy*. Canberra: Commonwealth Department of Health and Aged Care, 1999.

[38] Liamputtong P, Lin V, Bagley P. Ethnic communities and health reforms. In: H Gardner, P Liamputtong (eds.), *Health, Social Policy, and Communities*. Melbourne: Oxford University Press, 2002 (in press).

[39] Davis P, Beaglehole R, Durie M. Directions for public health in the new millennium. *NZ Pub Hlth Report* 2000; 7: 1–3, 10.

[40] Ellis PM, Collings SCD (eds.). *Mental Health in New Zealand from a Public Health Perspective*. Public Health Report number 3. Wellington: Ministry of Health, 1997.

Chapter 12

Bioterrorism: The extreme politics of public health

Richard Horton

YOU CANNOT STOP US. WE HAVE THIS ANTHRAX. YOU DIE NOW. ARE YOU AFRAID? DEATH TO AMERICA

This hand written letter was sent to the *New York Times* after the terrorist air attacks on New York and Washington, DC, on 11 September 2001 and after the first report of inhalational anthrax in Boca Raton, Florida. It was no mere threat. The index case of bioterrorism in the United States was Robert Stevens, a 63-year-old man who worked as a photo editor for a major tabloid newspaper. He died after a short and dramatic illness, which was initially misdiagnosed as bacterial meningitis [1].

The fear surrounding anthrax—no terrorist-associated case had been described in the United States before—understandably persuaded the clinicians looking after this man to defer a press announcement until local public health authorities had confirmed the diagnosis. There would be, in the words of the doctors involved, "serious ramifications" once such a disclosure was made. And there were. When the first report of this successful bioterrorist attack was released on 4 October, panic spread throughout the United States, and beyond. Anthrax was discovered in the building in which the man worked. Regional and local postal centers were scoured for traces of the organism and they too were positive.

Anthrax spores were found in letters within federal buildings, and the US government was forced to suspend some activities while offices were searched and decontaminated. Investigation of the postal facility handling government mail revealed that *Bacillus anthracis* had been dispersed in an aerosolised form, causing four further cases of inhalational anthrax, two of whom died.

These four individuals had handled letters arriving in Senate offices on 15 October [2,3]—letters that had been posted on 9 October. Despite public knowledge about the Florida index case, anthrax was not high on the list of differential diagnoses for doctors seeing these four later presentations. The two patients who subsequently died remained untreated for seven and five days, respectively. In all, there were five deaths from anthrax and eighteen nonfatal cases of this rare infection. A bioterrorist act had been highly effective: fear had paralysed much of the country and normal government business was disrupted.

Here was the first lesson for public health. Transfer of information from a surveillance input to a service output, via a central public health co-ordinating network, has to be fast—faster than the system seemed capable of achieving. Early diagnosis and treatment is likely to save lives [3]. A second lesson concerned the sensory capacity of the public health system. If the bioterrorist threat is to be resisted, then diagnostic facilities must be in place for proper appraisal of these rare but lethal infections. Finally, the entire medical community needs to educate itself about infections that could be vehicles for bioterrorist acts. For the first time in the history of the western world, biological agents need to be considered seriously in any patient presenting with an unusual or atypical illness. Rather chillingly, the scientific reality is that "only further experience with this devastating disease can clarify its precise natural history and optimal treatment". [3] Reviewers of this "new challenge for American medicine", wrote of a "new era" in their country's history of public health [4]. Fear had led well over 30,000 people to be treated pre-emptively with antibiotics because of concern about possible exposure to anthrax, emphasising the critical importance of distributing information through reputable (e.g., www.bt.cdc.gov) internet sites, not only for physicians but also for the public [4].

But the immediate and more important public health impact of these bioterrorist attacks was on psychological well-being. A measure of the likely effect was described in a national survey of stress reactions after the original 11 September air assaults [5]. Two in five adults surveyed described one or more symptoms of stress, such as feeling very upset on being reminded of the 11 September events; disturbed memories, thoughts, or dreams; difficulty concentrating; sleep disturbance; or irritable outbursts. These indicators of stress also affected children. The degree of anxiety seemed to be associated with television exposure to the terrorist incidents.

These events have had an instant effect on government research policy—and funding [6]. After an initial $5.1 billion was committed to bioterrorism defence and research in 2001, a further $11 billion was promised in 2002. This money will be spent on stockpiling vaccines and antibiotics, building new laboratories, funding basic research, and designing drug and vaccine discovery programs.

The European Union has also raised civil protection from biological attacks higher in its list of funding priorities, with special attention being given to detection and diagnosis, surveillance, vaccines, and pooling of knowledge between member states. Within the space of a few months, protecting the public health from bioterrorism has assumed a position of unparalleled political importance.

The public health politics of bioterrorism

One of the more tangible domestic responses to the 11 September attacks on America was the appointment of Governor Tom Ridge of Pennsylvania to head a new Office of Homeland Defence. By this manoeuvre, the US government had now officially designated itself as vulnerable, its borders breached by acts of catastrophic violence that were compounded by subsequent anthrax assaults. Security experts had long ago pointed out the lack of American preparedness for terrorism [7].

The political failure to devise systems to protect the public from terrorist, and especially bioterrorist, attack runs deep. A survey of 456 US cities with populations of greater than 100,000 revealed that a third did not have a terrorism response or prevention plan in place [8]. Half of all cities had no antiterrorism training. Most remarkably of all, and this survey was conducted after the 11 September attacks, 48 percent of cities had no intention to conduct an overall reassessment of their preparedness.

The lack of an effective antiterrorist plan produced a chaotic domestic response when terrorists did strike. Fear of biological and chemical attacks led the Federal Aviation Administration to bring about a temporary agricultural crisis by grounding crop-dusting aeroplanes. At least one of the 11 September hijackers had downloaded information from the internet about the aerial distribution of pesticides. And yet experts on weapons of mass destruction argued that these aircraft were far more likely to be used as flying bombs, carrying fuel rather than biological or chemical agents.

One domestic strategy was a financial war on terrorism. An effort to freeze terrorist assets included key figures in al-Qaeda—Osama Bin Laden's terrorist organization—and other groups that channelled money to the Taliban regime in Afghanistan. The effect of this response was highly symbolic—in the words of one US government official, "it sends a powerful signal to al-Qaeda that we know who they are, who their friends are, and who supports them financially" [9]. More importantly, this statement sent a signal to the American public that, despite the attacks on their major cities and fears of bioterrorism, the government knew exactly who its enemy was. This counterterrorist measure was designed as much to calm public nerves as it was to stop terrorism.

An emphasis on securing and parading reliable information about individual terrorists was clearly intended to recoup what had been seen as the CIA's greatest failure [10]. Since one of the goals of any terrorist operation is to induce a state of pervasive fear and anxiety among those who inhabit its target, countering that mental state must be a major antiterrorist strategy. This approach therefore becomes an important aspect of the public health response to terrorism: reducing mass public anxiety by offering reassurance that government has all the necessary intelligence to protect its people. Thought of in this way, the CIA has features of a public health agency as well as an intelligence service. Its failure is a public health failure as well as an intelligence failure, and its fundamental mistake was to create an information vacuum not only at the center of government but also among the public. But there is another interpretation of these events, one that has important implications for public health responses to bioterrorist threats—namely, that the failure to alert public and government alike to danger was not due to a lack of information but rather to ignored information. To see how an aversion to evidence creates the climate for inaction, one only has to look at recent US press and government responses to escalating terrorist threats [11]. On 7 August 1998, two US embassies in East Africa were bombed, killing over 200 people and injuring thousands. In retaliation, President Clinton authorized the bombing of a pharmaceutical manufacturing plant in Khartoum on 20 August 1998. The basis for the US attack was evidence of chemical weapons collected from a soil sample at the site of the plant. Yet this response was largely seen as Clinton's most serious foreign policy error, occurring at a time of intense public scrutiny of his personal integrity.

Al-Qaeda admitted responsibility for the bombings in Nairobi and Dar-es-Salaam. Evidence later secured from a witness in the trial of those responsible for these attacks lent support not only to Clinton's justification for the bombing but also to the pivotal role of al-Qaeda. The security services had gathered sufficient information to alert them to the threat from al-Qaeda. Given the evidence that Osama Bin Laden's network had acquired components for biological weapons, dismissal of a bioterrorist threat as an exaggerated overreaction was, with hindsight, complacent. The greatest danger to intelligence and public health agencies trying to protect citizens from biological attack is a climate of scepticism—even apathy—about the risks.

The perverse limitations of an open society when dealing with external threats to domestic security—a culture that supports individual rights enabling would-be terrorists to learn the skills they need to terrorize—have led to speculation about society's norms of tolerance and civilized behavior. An example was offered by *Newsweek* columnist, Jonathan Alter, who argued that it was "time to think about torture [of terrorist suspects] to jump-start the stalled investigation of the greatest crime in American history" [12]. Public health workers have an important role here in preventing abuses of human rights, irrespective of their ends and however justifiable they might seem.

But the most important political, and perhaps public health, consequence of the 11 September attacks and anthrax deaths has been a reassessment of America's place in world affairs. In order to build a coalition against terrorism, the United States has embarked on its biggest global diplomatic effort since the Cold War. In doing so, it forged alliances with countries that had previously been anathema to its foreign policy interests, notably Pakistan. For once, America needed the world on its side. A Republican government discarded its own isolationist policies to achieve its new aims. It will have to maintain that enlarged commitment to global co-operation if its war on terrorism is to succeed. In the long-term this stark shift in policy might have profound impact on US attitudes to issues that go beyond bioterrorism in their relevance to public health (e.g., climate change, development aid, environmental policy, and issues of international human rights and criminal law). President Bush's veto in July 2001 of a draft protocol adding enforcement and verification mechanisms to the 1972 Biological and Toxin Weapons Convention, which had prohibited the development, testing, production, and stockpiling of biological weapons, was an example of how US isolationism harmed not only global efforts to reduce terrorist threats but also homeland security. Will national sovereignty now come second to global security and public health? The early indications are that although the US government recognizes that there are global issues to be resolved, its own national interests (and international reputation as a superpower accountable to nobody but itself) will not be diluted by larger strategic or humanitarian concerns.

National responses to bioterrorism: A UK case study

The history of public health policy towards bioterrorist threats in the United Kingdom is one of the revisions and reversals [13]. The first fears began after a July 1934, report that German spies had tested biological agents on the London underground. This matter was viewed as a public health problem and referred to the UK's Medical Research Council.

By contrast with modern perspectives on bioterrorism, it was believed that a biological threat resided in the consequences of public health service disruptions caused by conventional warfare. A breakdown in sanitary services could leave many people vulnerable to crippling epidemics of infectious disease, for example, from the bacteria, especially tetanus, that cause wound infections. Anthrax and typhoid were also discussed. After a great deal of protracted committee debate, it was agreed that the time had come for an Emergency Public Health Laboratory Service (PHLS). Sparked by the threat of biological warfare seen through this broad public health perspective, the PHLS, established in 1947, today "protects the population from infection by detecting, diagnosing, and monitoring communicable diseases". It consists of a central public health laboratory, a communicable disease surveillance centre, and forty-six local laboratories.

With the advent of World War II, an explicit research effort into biological warfare was launched. By 1943, a prototype anthrax bomb had been built. The year 1947 saw biological weapons research achieve equal priority with nuclear research. Sea trials with pathogens took place up to the mid-1950s. But this offensive effort soon switched to more defensive goals when the military establishment eventually cancelled its order for a biological bomb. Although research continued, it has never reached the profile it had in the immediate post-war period.

After the Gulf War, politicians and scientists shared renewed interest in biological weapons. In 1999, the UK's Royal Society, together with the US National Academy of Sciences and French Academie des Sciences met to consider the control of biological agents [14]. The Royal Society's report urged "a scientifically sound and realistic assessment" of the effects of potential biological agents. They also recommended that medical staff should be trained to recognise diseases caused by biological weapons and that limited national vaccine banks and stockpiles of antibiotics should be created. Most importantly,

> "To manage the consequences of a biological weapons attack on civilians, an overall structure is needed within which attacks by specific agents can be handled. Collaborative plans should be set up between the police, public health authorities, the clinical and hospital services, the intelligence agencies and the military. The authorities who would co-ordinate the local and national responses should be made clear. These plans should be tested in simulated attacks."

None of these measures were implemented. Thus, when the UK Parliament's Defence Committee met in November 2001 to consider the threat from terrorism [15], there was little evidence to draw on for substantive public inquiry. Still, a crucial shift in policy emerged during this gathering of evidence:

> "In the past the level of resources put into the defence of the UK has been set principally to reflect the perceived level of threat rather than through an

assessment of the weak points in our society. Provisionally we have concluded that in the UK we will have to do more to focus our capabilities on defending our weak points."

The conclusion of the Defence Committee was that the threat of nonstate terrorism was increasing, especially concerning weapons of mass destruction. Bioterrorism is the greatest danger of all, although its effects are uncertain. Biological weapons are required in small quantities, are low cost, and have high strategic impact. They have the weakest international controls of any weapon. What limited evidence exists suggests that terrorist organizations are trying to secure biological materials. Presently, the United Kingdom could not respond to a large-scale terrorist attack. An urgent military review will be required, including an appraisal of homeland security and the place of the military in civilian protection.

The United Kingdom was judged unable to offer a unilateral program for homeland defence. Therefore, international institutions must act on behalf of their individual members to provide the necessary levels of domestic protection. NATO's decision to invoke Article five of its treaty (that an attack against one member country is an attack against all countries) on 12 September 2001, and UN Security Council Resolution 1373, passed on 28 September 2001, which declared that nations must deny safe haven to terrorist organizations and their supporters, are good examples of this co-ordinated international response.

When the Home Affairs Committee [16] took evidence to underpin the Anti-Terrorism, Crime and Security Act 2001 [17], there was a specific interest in protecting the public's health from bioterrorist threats. Politicians were most concerned with the need for a proportionate response and for care over constructing rules of detention without trial of suspected terrorists. The balance between protecting the public (health) and protecting individual rights was not easily achieved. Eventually, it was reluctantly agreed that detention when there was no prospect of extradition, deportation, or prosecution was allowable in rare circumstances. Provisions covering data sharing, racial and religious offences, hoaxers, powers of identification (e.g., fingerprinting), aviation security, police authority, and freezing financial assets were all covered in this latest Act.

But it was the bioterrorism-inspired PHLS that provided the immediate anchor for efforts to construct a practicable and responsive public health strategy. By 31 October 2001, less than a month after the first anthrax letter was opened in the United States, the PHLS had issued interim guidance for health professionals dealing with packages suspected of containing anthrax (see www.phls.co.uk). The advice begins with the comment that any threat of bioterrorism in the United Kingdom remained low. It acknowledged the genuine public anxiety about biological weapons and stated that the PHLS guidance was a proportionate response to this anxiety. Yet the advice, together with its implications, was strong; every business was recommended to review its protocols for handling mail.

In January 2002, the UK's Chief Medical Officer, Liam Donaldson, published a national strategy document for dealing with the threat of infectious disease [18]. This investigation had been long promised, but now took account of the risk posed by biological weapons. The report was withering in its criticism of anti-infection arrangements in the United Kingdom. There was no integrated approach to the problem of infectious disease; no clear lines of responsibility; no reliable infrastructure; no standardised diagnostic criteria for infections; and poor laboratory security procedures. To counter these profound weaknesses, Donaldson recommended the creation of a National Infection Control and Health Protection Agency. The threat from bioterrorism, he argued, had been judged low because of the technical difficulty of launching a biological attack. In the light of the terrorist attacks in the United States,

"The possibility of a much more extensive terrorist operation, the absence of a specific warning, the deployment of terrorists who have no fear for their personal safety or survival, and the use of multiple simultaneous points of attack must now form part of the planning for countermeasures to protect the health of the population against deliberate release."

His analysis ended with a recommendation that dealt directly with the central criticism of intelligence services in the US 11 post-September — namely, a failure of imagination. He advised "Forward thinking and innovation in identifying and protecting against vulnerability."

In sum, the anatomy of the public health response to the reality of bioterrorism is part medical and part political. The necessary public health measures to tackle biological weapons had been discussed before the October 2001, incidents in the United States. Government authorities, while paying lip service to this advice, did little to engage with these measures seriously. Since October 2001, that advice has been reiterated and enlarged—and money is at last moving to shore up public health defences (in the United States $1 billion for states to improve bioterrorism defences, and $3 billion for the Department of Health and Human Services to begin preparedness planning [ten times the department's budget in 2001]). But bioterrorism also substantially widens the scope of public health. By the very nature of the threat, protecting the public's health involves intelligence gathering, strengthening criminal justice, and reassessing defence and foreign policy initiatives. There are few contemporary issues that require such a broad conception—an extreme politics—of public health, yet public health has much to offer policy development in each area.

Medicine versus terrorism: Rhetoric or responsibility?

The response of the medical and scientific communities to the events of 11 September and subsequent anthrax attacks showed that doctors and scientists believe they have an important part to play in limiting the risks of bioterrorism. Public health has been described as "a kind of homeland defence that is applicable to both unintentional and intentional disease outbreaks" [19]; health-care workers were likely to be the first to respond to a biological attack and so disease surveillance, together with domestic and international networks for notification, were crucial defensive counter-terrorist measures. Senior scientists and administrators at the UK's Public Health Laboratory Service [20] drew attention to PHLS guidance on covert pathogen releases and wrote that the UK's "excellent public health systems and infrastructure give us a good start" in laying down a preventive system to combat bioterrorist threats.

The view that further biological weapons use is inevitable is now commonplace. Yet the equally common view is that countries are ill-prepared for a biological attack [21,22]. The fact that a biological incident would begin silently—no explosions, no warnings—makes effective preparation almost impossible. D A Henderson, now director of the Center for Civilian Biodefence at Johns Hopkins University, has argued that there is "no comprehensive national plan nor any agreed strategy for dealing with the problems of biological weapons". Antibiotic and vaccine stocks are simply inadequate to deal with such an attack. This impression was borne out by a study of disaster preparedness in New York City [23]. Fewer than two-thirds of directors of emergency receiving hospitals had protocols for dealing with biological attacks and only a third felt very or moderately confident about managing victims of a biological incident. Early mistakes by senior American politicians, for example, in failing to rely on health officials to act as key information sources for the public, seemed to bear out this uncertainty [24].

Yet the escalating threat of biological weapons had been predicted by the public health community. A US working group on civilian biodefence, supported by the Department of Health and Human Services' Office of Emergency Preparedness, had been publishing regular consensus statements on potential biological agents, such as anthrax [25], smallpox [26], plague [27], botulinum toxin [28], and tularaemia [29]. This careful process of defining the threat and drawing up guidance on diagnosis, vaccination, treatment, prophylaxis, and decontamination stemmed from the failure of the Biological Weapons and Toxin Convention to contain the threat successfully. The US Centers for Disease Control and Prevention played a critical part in strengthening public health defences [30], although a lack of ability to respond to surges in demand remained a serious weakness [31].

Moreover, once the first anthrax case was reported in October 2001, health officials quickly secured supplies of ciprofloxacin at reduced cost, after the US government put pressure on Bayer, the drug's manufacturer, to cut its price, even though other drugs are much cheaper and at least as effective. Scientists at the Centers for Disease Control and Prevention acted immediately to determine how the first patient contracted the disease and which genetic strains of *B anthracis* were used. Thus, while it might be true that "The nation has short-sightedly allowed its public health agencies and facilities to weaken in recent years", [32] it is also true to say that those same agencies acted remarkably quickly and effectively to deal with the threat once it became real.

Some critics might argue that the US government has reacted too quickly. Is it appropriate, for example, for the government to accelerate safety trials of a new smallpox vaccine? Drug companies are being asked to rush through clinical trials to have a vaccine available by the end of 2002 [33]. Can safety reasonably be marginalized in the interests of national security? And, in any case, at what cost to other social programs? The increases in US bioterrorism budgets have forced a rebalancing of welfare priorities—services for the elderly and uninsured are likely to be cut, and CDC's nonbioterrorism spending will fall with likely adverse effects on public health generally.

Each country will have its own administrative and scientific resources to design national public health policies on bioterrorism. But there is also scope for co-ordinated regional planning. The anthrax attacks in the United States led to further calls for "a centralised structure" within Europe "to co-ordinate advanced research, surveillance and professional training". [34] Although this idea remains little more than a well-argued concept agreed upon by a small group of enthusiasts, the shared police resources and enhanced European co-operation post-September 11 may rekindle the idea among national politicians.

What can those concerned with public health achieve globally? In 1997, Joshua Lederberg argued that "The medical community does indeed have a primary role in institutionalizing the prohibition of biological weapons as a global commandment, as well as in mitigating the harm from infractions." [35] At *The Lancet*, we argued that this international imperative could be achieved through a new global coalition against terror [36]. But we cautioned that

> "For many nations that were born out of what was once labelled terrorism, efforts to eradicate totally a method of protest that was part of their own historic political struggle are likely to be resisted ... Diplomacy will be confronted by histories that cannot be separated from politics."

Still, public health—through ideas such as harm reduction, human rights, population approaches to health, and social medicine—has a central role in disarming the terrorist: "Attacking hunger, disease, poverty, and social exclusion might do more good than air marshals, asylum restrictions, and identity cards" [37]. Transnational communities of doctors, scientists, and other professionals can do much to foster tolerance between countries [38]. Medicine acts as a bridge between societies since it sets out shared concerns for prevention, care, and healing [39]. These principles have been shown to have powerful effects during wars and their aftermath [40]. The World Medical Association has called for the creation of an international consortium of medical and public health leaders to monitor the threat of biological weapons, to identify actions to stop bioweapons proliferation, and to develop a plan for monitoring the world wide emergence of infectious diseases. All that is now lacking is leadership to convert these ideas into reality. Furthermore, public health approaches to counterterrorism cannot ignore the development debate. Terrorism breeds in collapsed states, although many recent terrorists have come from the educated middle classes of Saudi Arabia. The conditions for state failure are a mix of poverty, disease, inequality, debt, poor infrastructure, lack of effective administrative capacity, weak governance, and state violence. Public health therefore has a political, economic, and social, as well as a medical, agenda to follow. Constructing or rebuilding health services in poor nations—e.g., Afghanistan—is one practical consequence. Each individual within the public health community can take part in shaping this agenda. Perhaps there is even a duty to take part.

The most radical opportunity for the public health community to develop this role came with the report published in 2001 by the Commission on Macroeconomics and Health [41]. The Commission was established by WHO's Director-General, Gro Harlem Brundtland, in 2000. Its aim was to place the health of the poor at the centre of the development agenda. The argument underpinning this effort was that disease is inherently destabilising for economies and entire political systems. The stability of the global economy depends, therefore, on an effective program to reduce disease burdens and improve the health of the poorest people. The Commission concluded that by focusing on only a few diseases—e.g., TB, malaria, and HIV–AIDS—eight million lives per year could be saved by 2010. At a total annual cost of $66 billion ($34 per person per year in low-to-middle income countries) the economic benefit could be $360 billion per year by 2020. Present donor contributions are about $6 billion per year. That figure must increase to $27 billion per year by 2007 if these benefits are to be realized. If one accepts the twin assumptions that investing in health will bring political stability and economic development, and that state failure fosters terrorism, investment in health may be an important counterterrorist measure. Whether the causal chain for terrorism is so simple remains to be seen, of course.

Historical evidence complicates this analysis by pointing to the waves of political repression that can force moderate opposition groups to adopt more extreme—and violent—positions in countries that may not be failing. For example, Ahmed Rashid has argued that the oppression of moderate Islamic political parties in central Asia during an era of Soviet influence produced terrorist groups that remain active and a threat to the western world today [42].

Information or propaganda?

Is the threat of bioterrorism illusory? Simon Wesseley and colleagues have claimed that the main purpose of biological weapons "is to wreak destruction via psychological means—by inducing fear, confusion, and uncertainty in everyday life" [43]. They argue that the long-term psychological and social consequences of the threat are likely to be more serious than the physical risk itself. Their argument is not new [44]. However, our experience with anthrax is too little to make such confident assurances. The fact is that biological weapons have been made, are being designed, and are likely to be used again. The accidental outbreak of anthrax in the Soviet Union on 2 April 1979, which caused at least sixty-six deaths, showed that this agent was being prepared within a military facility in a country that had signed an international agreement not to do so [45]. The risk of bioterrorism is credible.

From a public health perspective, therefore, the key means of protection is good surveillance [46]. One approach that might amplify the ability to report, confirm, or prevent outbreaks is the use of the internet as a means of civil defence [47]. Ronald Laporte and colleagues believe that the "existing international public health system is not sufficiently agile to compete with bioterrorists". They advocate devolving surveillance to citizens who would become "the first and most important line of defence". The capacity of the public health system would expand enormously, fear might be averted by sharing responsibility among a larger community, and the necessary communication network would also double as an effective mechanism for distributing information. This argument has been implicitly accepted by US government agencies. The FBI sent half a million letters to New Jersey and Pennsylvania residents inviting their help in identifying the anthrax assailant. "Look at your neighbour and see if he fits this profile", one postal inspector said [48].

Indeed, the failure to pass on accurate information to the public about the anthrax incident showed how weak and unreliable public health systems of communication really are [49]. When news of the first anthrax case was initially reported, instead of acknowledging the possibility of bioterrorism, admitting uncertainty, and reassuring the public that the incident was urgently being investigated, US Health and Human Services Secretary Tommy Thompson described the case as one of natural origin with no evidence of underlying terrorism. The most authoritative agency in the nation able to give advice on bioterrorism—the CDC—was silenced on the grounds that an anthrax attack was within criminal not public health jurisdiction. No consistent message was given by a respected and reliable public health source.

But when does information become propaganda? The front cover of the 6 October 2001, *Economist* ran the headline, "The Propaganda War". The editors were referring to the US Government's need to tell its story about its motives and future plans for attacking Afghanistan. But propaganda also refers to the talking up and talking down of the bioterrorist threat. The immediate government response was to talk the threat down. Result: that when a case of anthrax was confirmed, there was widespread and unnecessary fear. Either the government did not have a grip on the situation or it was being complacent.

This response shows how dangerous it is when governments mistrust public reaction. It shows that the dominant view, even in democratic societies, is that public information must be kept tightly controlled. One manifestation of this overmanagement is the political effort in both the United States and United Kingdom to suppress full scientific reporting of allegedly sensitive research work. Such restrictions are perhaps understandable in the wake of 11 September. But they usher in an era of censorship and the closure of previously open institutions and disciplines. This precedent threatens not only centuries-old free exchange of scientific ideas but also the wider rights of free expression won by democracies worldwide [50]. Taking a phrase from the American journalist, Walter Lippmann, Noam Chomsky has referred to this media management as "manufacturing consent" [51]. Consent, that is, for the prevailing government policy of the day. It is perilous, to speculate on the motive behind the initial Thompson denial. Certainly, he would have wished that what he said was true. But maybe also, since there was nothing the government could do about an anthrax attack, his immediate denial bought the government time, and masked national impotence.

There is one final question that remains unanswered. Who sent the letters laced with anthrax? By late 2002, the FBI had failed to find the perpetrators. The reward for public information about the attacks rose to $2.5 million. There is no proof that the origin was an al-Qaeda cell within the United States. The terrorist might reasonably have been an opportunist. Or, like Timothy McVeigh, the Oklahoma bomber, a right-wing anarchist. The anthrax incident poses a serious problem for the US government, indeed all governments. The bioterrorist threat may not only be from within US borders, but also from US citizens. There is evidence that lax procedures and poor security at the US Army's Fort Detrick biowarfare research centre might have provided the opportunity for a revenge attack by a disgruntled employee. Stricter laboratory security procedures are being implemented, but quietly. This is not a line of inquiry the US government particularly wishes to debate, since it would blunt its efforts to secure an international coalition to fight terrorists outside US borders.

Indeed, the US government's slogan—a "war against terrorism"—serves the immediate political purpose of retaliation for the appalling atrocities of 11 September. But it also drives attention away from a wider and less politically acceptable issue—namely, that to stop terrorism demands rescuing failed states from oblivion and responding to the challenge of political repression and increasing social and economic inequalities. That means national and personal financial, even human, sacrifice for a cause that neither the government nor the wider public may see as immediately relevant to US interests.

The ultimate answer for the public health community—incorporating, as it does, the most extreme definition of public health's reach—lies in working to promote an open society, one based on understanding a country's place and responsibilities in world affairs. One of the more optimistic outcomes of 11 September was the decision by US national news networks to expand their overseas news coverage after decades of attrition [52].

The task for public health practitioners is two-fold. First, to put in place effective systems for dealing with a bioterrorist attack. Foresight planning and surveillance are key. Food supplies, for example, remain a worrying vulnerability [53]. In the United States in 1984, a religious cult successfully contaminated salad bars with *Salmonella typhimurium*. The centralised production and complex distribution of much of America's food makes it an easy target for determined terrorists. Botulism might well be their preferred weapon. Second, the public health community must help to create the conditions for prevention. Most importantly, that means working beyond national borders to support the many shared values among different peoples—dignity, respect, compassion, trust—which emphasise our common human purpose.

WHO has taken an important lead. After a new resolution on the global public health response to biological, chemical, and nuclear material was adopted at the May, 2002, World Health Assembly [54], WHO has assisted member countries in devising national plans for public health preparedness. Most resources have been directed into surveillance and early warning systems. The agency has also helped create networks of experts and institutions for the potentially most threatening diseases e.g., smallpox and anthrax. In the aftermath of the terrorist attacks on the United States, much was made of a clash of civilizations—Islam versus the West. Yet not only is this dichotomy naive, it is antithetical to all the traditions of inclusiveness that mark public health as a truly social discipline. Bioterrorism provides a compelling example of why those concerned with the public's health must rediscover their passion for radical engagement with international affairs, if broad public health goals are to be achieved.

References

[1] Bush LM, Abrams BH, Beall A, Johnson CC. Index case of fatal inhalational anthrax due to bioterrorism in the US. *N Engl J Med* 2001; **345**: 1607–10.

[2] Borio L, Frank D, Mani V et al. Death due to bioterrorism-related inhalational anthrax. *JAMA* 2001; **286**: 2554–59.

[3] Mayer TA, Bersoff-Matcha S, Murphy C et al. Clinical presentation of inhalational anthrax following bioterrorism exposure. *JAMA* 2001; **286**: 2549–53.

[4] Lane HC, Fauci AS. Bioterrorism on the home front. *JAMA* 2001; **286**: 2595–97.

[5] Schuster MA, Stein BD, Jaycox LH et al. A national survey of stress reactions after the September 11, 2001, terrorist attacks. *N Engl J Med* 2001; **345**: 1507–12.

[6] Marcus J, Nuthall K. Researchers join war on terror. *Times Higher Education* (Supplement) January 4, 2002: 1.

[7] Nye JS. How to protect the homeland? *New York Times*, September 25, 2001: A29.

[8] Caffrey A, Gold R. Before Federal security office forms, states get a jump on defenses. *Wall Street Journal*, September 25, 2001: A6.

[9] Miller J. The 27 whose assets will be frozen are just the first of many, a US official says. *New York Times*, September 25, 2001: B4.

[10] Hersh SM. What went wrong. *New Yorker*, October 8, 2001: 34–40.

[11] Benjamin D, Simon S. A failure of intelligence? *New York Review of Books*, December 20, 2001: 76–80.

[12] Alter J. Time to think about torture. *Newsweek*, November 5, 2001.

[13] Balmer B. *Britain and biological warfare*. Basingstoke: Palgrave, 2001.

[14] The Royal Society. *Measures for Controlling the Threat from Biological Weapons*. London: Royal Society, 2000.

[15] Defence Committee. *The Threat from Terrorism*, Vols. I and II. London: Stationery Office, 2001.

[16] Home Affairs Committee. *The Anti-Terrorism, Crime and Security Bill 2001*. London: Stationery Office, 2001.

[17] *Anti-Terrorism, Crime and Security Act 2001*. London: Stationery office, 2001.

[18] Chief Medical Officer. *Getting Ahead of the Curve: A Strategy for Combating Infectious Diseases*. London: Department of Health, 2001.

[19] Chyba CF. Biological security in a changed world. *Science* 2001; **293**: 2349.

[20] Lightfoot N, Wale M, Spencer R, Nicoll A. Appropriate responses to bioterrorist threats. *BMJ* 2001; **323**: 877–78.

[21] Simon JD. Biological terrorism: preparing to meet the threat. *JAMA* 1997; **278**: 428–30.

[22] Flam F. US is poorly prepared for a biological attack. *The Philadelphia Inquirer*. September 25, 2001: 1.

[23] Silber SH, Oster N, Simmons B, Garrett C. Y2K medical disaster preparedness in New York City. *Prehosp Disast Med* 2001; **16**: 88–95.

[24] Pear R. In anthrax crisis, health secretary finds unsteady going. *New York Times*. October 25, 2001.

[25] Inglesby TV, Henderson DA, Bartlett JG et al. Anthrax as a biological weapon: Medical and public health management. *JAMA* 1999; **281**: 1735–45.

[26] Henderson DA, Inglesby TV, Bartlett JG et al. Smallpox as a biological weapon: Medical and public health management. *JAMA* 1999; **281**: 2127–37.

[27] Inglesby TV, Henderson DA, Bartlett JG et al. Plague as a biological weapon: Medical and public health management. *JAMA* 1999; **283**: 2281–90.

[28] Arnon SS, Schechter R, Inglesby TV et al. Botulinum toxin as a biological weapon: Medical and public health management. *JAMA* 2001; **285**: 1059–70.

[29] Dennis DT, Inglesby TV, Henderson DA et al. Tularemia as a biological weapon: Medical public health management. *JAMA* 2001; **285**: 2763–73.

[30] Khan AS, Morse S, Lillibridge S. Public-health preparedness for biological terrorism in the USA. *Lancet* 2000; **356**: 1179–82.

[31] O'Toole T, Inglesby TV. Facing the biological weapons threat. *Lancet* 2000; **356**: 1128–29.

[32] Editorial. The spector of biological terror. *New York Times*. September 26, 2001.

[33] Denny C. Rules relaxed in rush for new smallpox vaccine. *The Guardian*. October 25, 2001.

[34] Tibayrenc M. A European centre to respond to threats of bioterrorism and major epidemics. *Bull WHO* 2001; **79**: 1094.

[35] Lederberg J. Infectious disease and biological weapons: prophylaxis and mitigation. *JAMA* 1997; **278**: 435–36.

[36] Editorial. A world war against terrorism. *Lancet* 2001; **358**: 937–38.

[37] Horton R. Public health: a neglected counterterrorist measure. *Lancet* 2001; **58**: 1112–13.

[38] Horton R. Violence and medicine: the necessary politics of public health. *Lancet* 2001; **358**: 1472–73.

[39] MacQueen G, Santa-Barbara J, Neufeld V, Yusuf S, Horton R. Health and peace: Time for a new discipline. *Lancet* 2001; **357**: 1460–61.

[40] Horton R. Croatia and Bosnia: The imprints of war-II. Restoration. *Lancet* 1999; **353**: 2223–28.

[41] Commission on Macroeconomics and Health. *Macroeconomics and Health: Investing in Health for Economic Development*. Geneva: World Health Organisation, 2001.

[42] Rashid A. *Jihad: The Rise of Militant Islam in Central Asia*. New Haven: Yale University Press, 2002.

[43] Wesseley S, Hyams KC, Bartholomew R. Psychological implications of chemical and biological weapons. *BMJ* 2001; **323**: 878–79.

[44] Holloway HC, Norwood AE, Fullerton CS, Engel CC, Ursano RJ. The threat of biological weapons. *JAMA* 1997; **278**: 425–27.

[45] Maselson M, Guillemin J, Hugh-Jones M et al. The Sverdlovsk anthrax outbreak of 1979. *Science* 1994; **266**: 1202–08.

[46] Geberding JL, Hughes JM, Koplan JP. Bioterrorism preparedness and response. *JAMA* 2002; **287**: 898–900.

[47] LaPorte RE, Sauer F, Dearwater S et al. Towards an internet civil defence against bioterrorism. *The Lancet Infectious Diseases* 2001; **1**: 125–27.

[48] Burkeman O. Anthrax reward soars as FBI draw a blank. *The Guardian.* January 26, 2002, 17.

[49] Altman LK, Kolata G. Anthrax missteps offer guide to fight next bioterror battle. *New York Times.* January 6, 2002.

[50] Editorial. A backhanded assault on academic freedom. *Lancet* 2002; **359**: 874–80.

[51] Chomsky N. *Media control: the spectacular achievements of propaganda*. New York: Seven Stories, 1997.

[52] Rutenberg J. Networks move to revise foreign news. *New York Times.* September 24, 2001: **C10**.

[53] Sobel J, Khan AS, Swerdlow DL. Threat of a biological terrorist attack on the US food supply: the CDC perspective. *Lancet* 2002; **359**: 874–80.

[54] WHO's response to that threat of the deliberate use of biological and chronical agents to cause harm. *Weekly Epidemiological Record* 2002; **77**: 281–87.

Chapter 13

Ethical issues in global public health

Daniel Wikler and Richard Cash

Introduction

Ethical dilemmas arise at almost every turn in the practice of global public health, for example:

- Those who would save lives through public health measures must decide which lives to save.

- Interventions usually protect health, but because they sometimes carry risks, the claims of those who might be harmed must be heard.

- Those who intervene and those who are affected may have different preferences and values.

- Public health programmes sometimes require compromises with values such as privacy and liberty.

- Public health requires research involving human subjects, but there is an incomplete consensus on the social contract between subjects, scientists, sponsors, and society.

- The pursuit of global public health takes place in an unjust world, demanding its practitioners judge when and to what extent to compromise their ideals and standards in order to remain effective.

- Practitioners of public health must sometimes choose between the objectives and interests of the communities they serve, the donors and sponsors, and themselves.

This chapter surveys a few of these ethical quandaries as stimulus to consideration of ethical dimensions of global public health. After some general remarks on ethics, we take up: ethical issues encountered in global public health practice; ethical dimensions of health resource allocation; and ethical issues in research involving human subjects.

Our goal is to identify ethical issues that bear further reflection. We leave the task of proposing standards and solutions to others [1].

Responsibilities and values

Ethical issues are those involving actions and policies that are right or wrong, fair or unfair, just or unjust. There is no consensus on methods for resolving ethical dilemmas and controversies [2]. Nevertheless, we cannot escape ethical dilemmas, and we need to reason our way through them.

In view of the importance of health, the severity of suffering from the burden of disease, and the numbers of individuals involved, few fields of professional activity face ethical choices as potentially momentous as those encountered in public health. A decision to emphasize prevention of HIV infection over cure of AIDS in the poorest countries, for example, would affect the lives of millions. There are multiple agents involved, both individual and collective, including organizations, professions, and nations. In addition to having conflicting interests, these agents may not accept the same sets of moral rules.

Whose responsibility?

Only the cooperative effort of individuals, local and national agencies, the private sector, and donors and governments can protect global public health. All agree on this general proposition, but not on the actual assignment of responsibility to the respective agents. For example:

1. Some donors will expect even the poorest countries to offer something by way of health services to their citizens, and to give guarantees that donated funds will be used effectively. Should countries that do not meet this requirement lose donor support?

2. High prices stand in the way of access to many needed pharmaceuticals in poor countries. The marginal cost of producing many of these drugs is minimal, and when price barriers reduce sales, the result is continued suffering but no profits. By ordinary moral calculations, the case for providing these drugs in the poorest countries at cost or even for free is overwhelming [3]. But as publicly owned, for-profit enterprises, the primary responsibility of the drug manufacturers is to stockholders.

3. While all who suffer from disease deserve the sympathy of others, some assign responsibility to individuals to take elementary precautions. If properly educated, then individuals may be able to avoid HIV/AIDS and reduce the risk of diabetes, cancer, and cardiovascular disease. Should aid, whether from national governments or from foreign donors, be made conditional on individuals' assuming this responsibility? The public health significance of this question is great. For example, the World

Health Organization (WHO) has been criticized for placing tobacco control high on its agenda, on the grounds that this is a matter of individual choice over which public health authorities should have no authority [4].

4. Sponsors of health research in developing countries offer benefits to the host community that go beyond any treatment offered in the course of the investigation. In the past sponsors had no obligations to host communities beyond the standard protections offered to the participants themselves. But ethics advisory agencies have urged that sponsors of research be required to demonstrate that any treatments proven effective by research in developing countries be useful to and accessible by those who live there [5].

In these and other cases, the outcomes turn on economics and politics; but ethical judgment is also at issue. Refusing to aid countries that do not provide for their own citizens punishes individuals for the failings of their governments. Addiction to tobacco generally occurs before the age of majority [6] and this counts strongly against the claim that tobacco control is not a legitimate public health function. Requiring sponsors to become donors to health systems could make research on tropical diseases unaffordable. These considerations point to the substantive ethical debate needed in assigning responsibility.

Ethical considerations may motivate less than self-interest. Rich nations fear that infectious diseases may cross borders. Drug companies can reap rewards from public approval when they donate their products. Ethical deliberation is not necessarily to determine how to increase altruism, though that would be a favorable outcome, but to locate benchmarks of moral adequacy against which self-interested behavior can be evaluated.

Whose values?

Whose values should guide those who face ethical dilemmas in the course of public health work? Deference to the values of the community may enhance acceptance and compliance with public health advice. But public health workers can sometimes benefit communities by insisting on compliance with nontraditional norms and values, as in the condemnation of female circumcision, endorsement of the use of condoms to prevent the spread of sexually transmitted diseases, and refusing to abide by cultural norms that accord inferior status or stigma to women, sex workers, homosexuals and to lower castes.

Fortunately, moral beliefs are universal more often than not: every culture champions the honest, the selfless, and the brave, and disdains those who are corrupt, insensitive, selfish, or untrustworthy. Marked variation tends to cluster in certain domains, such as family, reproduction, and sex. What sometimes presents itself as a difference in moral beliefs may, on analysis, simply reflect different understandings of scientific facts. These differences may be difficult to bridge, but they do not require a choice between one moral outlook and another [7].

Conflict might be resolvable by reference to international treaties, including human rights conventions, that have been ratified by the government of the host community, or by codes or guidelines of reputable professional societies or international organizations. The latter are sometimes devised specifically to protect the practitioner's freedom to act according to conscience in the face of pressure. A recent example is the proposed convention on "dual loyalties" for health professionals, drafted by Physicians for Human Rights, designed to reinforce health workers' dedication to the well-being of their patients regardless of the demands of state security agencies or employers [8]. Global conventions do not resolve the tension between conflicting moralities, since those who write these guidelines must decide whether they are to protect or to override the sovereignty of local authorities on these issues. They can, however, remove the burden of decision from the practitioner in the field.

Ethical issues in public health practice

The ethics of public health practice are based, as in clinical medicine, on the same fundamental principle of professional dedication to the best interests of the clients. The ethics of public health differ, however, in many ways. Public health takes into consideration the interests of the group or society as a whole, even when this may conflict with the best interests of some individuals [9]. In the case of global public health, the potential reach across national, cultural, and economic boundaries adds moral complexity. The moral requirement of informed consent creates problems in public health, both in terms of what constitutes genuine consent and in terms of who may be authorized to provide consent. In many countries, individual self-determination ranks high among the values governing the practice of medicine. This may not extend to public health, which must address conflicting needs of different parties and may rely on the power of the state to implement its recommendations. Public health workers often conduct surveillance of health conditions in the population that is not intrinsically linked to therapy or prevention for any individual patient, an activity which sometimes frustrates expectations on the part of sufferers. Indeed, research and monitoring must be built into public health interventions, since they may have serious unintended and harmful consequences (Box 13.1).

Box 13.1 Unintended consequences of public health interventions: arsenic in tube wells

For the past twenty-five years there has been a major effort to improve rural standards of water and hygiene in Bangladesh. The installation of tube wells has been the most important element of the programme with over 95 percent of the population now relying on groundwater from tube wells for drinking. Control of cholera and other water-borne enteric diseases was the stated purpose of increasing the availability of tube wells, though these wells were not routinely tested for microbial counts, heavy metals content, or toxic chemicals. In 1985, a physician in west Bengal, India began noticing patients with clinical signs of arsenic intoxication. (High levels of arsenic ingestion are associated with skin pigmentation and increased rates of a variety of cancers.) A check of tube wells revealed arsenic levels that were many times the recommended levels. As these areas bordered Bangladesh, authorities were informed but neither the government nor international donors, who had contributed significantly to tube well construction, took serious action. A national program has identified areas of high arsenic concentrations in tube well water; one-quarter of the population, or about thirty million people, are drinking water with significantly high levels of arsenic. Possible strategies to lower arsenic intake from water include: treating water at the pump; in-home treatment of water; community level water treatment; sealing wells with high arsenic content and returning to the use of treated surface water or collected rain water; and sinking deeper wells below the water table with high arsenic content. All these interventions are either costly or require continuing of maintenance. Some NGO's have mounted programs to reduce arsenic levels locally; however, there has been no national program to reduce tube well arsenic levels.

References

Smith AH, Lingas EO, Rahman M. Contamination of drinking-water by arsenic in Bangladesh: A public health emergency. *Bull WHO* 2000; 78: 1093–3.

Combating a Deadly Menace: Early Experience with a Community-Based Arsenic Mitigation Project in Bangladesh, Research Monograph Series No. 16, BRAC Research and Evaluation Division, Dhaka Bangladesh, August 2000.

Individuals and groups

The long-standing dilemma of choosing between individual and group interests in public health practice is most clearly at stake in the case of infectious disease epidemics. When, for public health reasons, commerce, travel, and personal relationships are disrupted, some individuals may suffer losses that exceed any protective benefits. These dilemmas arise regardless of who is given authority to protect the public's health. Reporting requirements for sexually transmitted diseases may benefit the general population, but weigh heavily on the individual. Vaccination, while generally safe, can impose risks that the child's parents might prefer to avoid if neighboring children accept the vaccines. In this case, it is in the best interest of each child to be the single individual who is not vaccinated.

Public health practitioners in the past sought to minimize these conflicts by ensuring that individuals receive proper attention even as populations were protected. For example, safer vaccinations reduce the risk to children, and strong guarantees of confidentiality minimize the social harm caused by contact tracing in STDs. But where the conflicts were unavoidable, the conventional public health view of ethics, unlike that of the individual physician, accepted the claims of the group. Perhaps this stance contributed to the success of public health over the past century in reducing mortality and morbidity. But it has also been blamed for contributing a moral outlook that was vulnerable to state-backed interventions in the name of the public's health. Mass sterilization and even murder in the eugenics movement of 1890–1950 [10] can be understood to reflect this view.

Tension between the interests of the group and the individual remains central to public health practice. Cuba's success in limiting the impact of sexually transmitted HIV/AIDS, for example, stemmed from a decision to subject individuals at risk to testing and to segregate those infected with the disease from the general population [11]. Contemporary developments in the ethics of public health suggest an alternative approach to this conflict that puts individual rights at its center [12]. In this view, individual human rights are key to preventing infection because spread of disease was facilitated by their denial. For example, women in many affected countries cannot refuse demands for unprotected sex. A second link to individual rights stemmed from the fact that the behavior that put individuals most at risk, including unsafe sex and the illicit use of unsanitary needles in drug abuse, took place in private, beyond the reach of the state. Only by assuring the individuals that their interests would be protected could they be recruited to join in a public health effort by modifying their behavior. In effect, the rights-centered approach to HIV infection required recognition of individual rights both on the basis of principle and also because, in this instance, this strategy was likely to be effective. But not all agree that expedience and principle coincide for HIV/AIDS, and have expressed concern over the idea that a rights-based approach partially absolves government of a complete commitment to an aggressive public health strategy [13].

Focusing on prevention

The emphasis on prevention that partially distinguishes public health from clinical medicine gives rise to further ethical difficulties. Health may be the highest priority for the public health practitioner, but not for many in the population who may reject intervention on their behalf as paternalistic [14]. Moreover, individuals vary in their perception of risk, and may be reluctant to accept the need for sacrificing liberties or changing lifestyles as the public health practitioner recommends [15]. In the case of pre-scientific populations in poor countries, the gap in knowledge and perception may be much wider. The potential exists for distrust, or conversely for excessive trust (at the expense of meaningful deliberation) [16]. Public health practitioners may find an ally in political authorities that claim to speak for their fellow-citizens and can order compliance, thus increasing acceptance but possibly at the expense of norms of self-determination. Public support for preventive measures that impose burdens of cost and loss of liberty is less certain when those who benefit and those who pay the price are not the same individuals. This is an issue inherent in public health prevention, in which the lives saved are "statistical": no one can know which individuals would have been afflicted had the prevention not have occurred. Rescue, whether of a child from a well or a patient needing expensive surgery, addresses the needs of "identi-fied" lives that attract the sympathy of all [17]. The arguable result is a persistent misallocation of resources away from preventive public health in the direction of curative clinical services.

Issues in health promotion

In all countries attempts to change health-related behavior on a mass scale face numerous ethical problems, whether the chosen means are communica-tion, incentives, coercion, or some combination. Although taxes on cigar-ettes are known to be an effective instrument in reducing the toll taken by tobacco [18], the individual's own calculation of the relative gain and loss may be different from that of the public health practitioner. Residents of the American state of Nevada, who have some of the least healthy living habits in the country, may look across the state line at their pious, clean-living neighbors in Utah and decide that, on the whole, they prefer the lifestyle they already enjoy (though, statistically speaking, they will not enjoy it as long) [19].

Some public health strategies for changing unhealthy lifestyles aim to identify those most at risk and to concentrate on reducing their personal risk factors. Other strategies aim to reduce risk for the population as a whole [20]. Both strategies face ethical dilemmas. Focusing on high-risk individuals, besides being expensive, risks stigmatizing the high-risk individuals, with possible consequences for employability and even social relationships. The population-wide strategy, which may be more affordable, seeks behavioral changes in individuals who might have remained healthy without them.

First, do no harm

To contrast the ethical norms governing public health and the generally accepted principles of clinical medicine, compromise or adaptation seems to be necessary on two fundamental tenets: doing no harm, and ensuring that the individual always decides. When public health interventions act in the interest of the group, some individuals may lose. Fortifying flour sold in food stores with folic acid, for example, reduces neural tube defects among newborns, but at the same time may mask the symptoms of vitamin deficiency in older people that would have prompted them to seek medical attention [21]. The practice of clinical medicine would be impossible if physicians were prevented from inducing harm in their patients under all circumstances, since medical care often involves risk-taking. The difference is that in the case of public health the risks are borne by some and the benefits may be enjoyed by others; there is of course no "body politic" akin to the body of the individual patient for whom losses for some individuals are compensated by gains to others, as harm to some of a given patient's cells may strengthen the patient overall.

Moreover, the ethics of risk must take account of the local environment. What represents too great a risk for one population may be a good bet for another. For example, a vaccine for rotavirus was withdrawn from the American market recently after several dozen children were found to have suffered from an intestinal disorder attributed to the vaccine. In the United States, children rarely die from rotavirus; the benefit of the vaccine was in preventing hospitalizations and the discomfort of diarrhea. In some developing countries, rotavirus is a leading cause of death for small children. The vaccine would remain an excellent choice in these countries, at least for poorer segments of the population that face the highest risk from diarrhoea [22]. Yet regulatory authorities were reluctant to approve the vaccine, fearful that the public would protest that a vaccine judged unsafe for American children was judged to be safe enough for them. This seemed, to some, to be a double standard of care, a violation of ethical rules in public health. Alternatively, the regulatory authorities might have reasoned that in the case of global public health what is owed to each child is care that has an optimal benefit-risk ratio. Given the large differences in risk level posed by rotavirus in poor and rich countries, application of this rule would yield different practices in different countries [23]. None of these issues can be resolved simply by reference to the rule of first do no harm.

Surveillance versus care

Basic epidemiological data are lacking in most poor countries, hampering the development of effective public health strategies. Public health workers who collect these data must make ethical choices between their primary mission and the inevitable demands from sick individuals whom they may encounter for personal health care. Provision of services would take time away from data collection and could render the data unrepresentative, undermining the rationale for stationing observers in the first place.

In some cases reasonable compromises may be very difficult to achieve. The WHO has been concerned over the possibility that disease may be spread in vaccination and other public health interventions due to the improper re-use of needles and inadequate sterilization of syringes. Observation of injection practices is indispensable if the authorities are to know whether the intervention does more good than harm. But what should the observer do if she sees that an individual is about to receive an unsafe injection? Intervening so that it does not take place would likely skew the data; indeed, intervention might result in the observer's being asked to leave at once. To stand by and say nothing would seem unconscionable to many, and could damage the good name of the health agency. WHO elected to intervene in all such cases.

Ethical dimensions of resource allocation

Public health interventions benefit some and not others. Choosing who will benefit requires ethics as much as it does economics and science. Attention to the ethics of public health resource allocation, particularly in international contexts, has only recently been undertaken [24]. The starting point for resource allocation in global public health is cost-effectiveness. The most cost-effective interventions yield the greatest gains in health per unit of cost. Ordinarily, the rule for allocation is maximization, which means choosing the most cost-effective mix of interventions available.

Conceptualizing, measuring, and calculating cost-effectiveness, and allocation strategies based on cost-effectiveness allocation, is complex and involves numerous ethical judgments [25]. Deciding what counts as a cost and how to measure health gains requires choosing between competing goods. The overall economic loss to a society when a productive or wealthy person becomes ill may be greater than when illness befalls a poor person, but we may decide to exclude these differences in cost so as to avoid counting the health and life of one person as being more valuable than the other [26]. Measuring health gains, too, involves a series of value-laden assumptions and decisions. We might seek to avoid making moral choices by asking the community to rank health losses; but this, too, is a moral choice. We might even choose to disregard these polls when they seem to reflect bias or stigma.

A maximizing strategy based on measures of cost-effectiveness makes resources go as far as possible, but the resulting allocation might conflict with ordinary notions of fairness [27]. People who are already well off may get the most benefit from a given health resource. For example, professional men who have access to health care and who can and do comply with physician advice may show more benefit in a hypertension treatment programme than poor, unemployed men living in a slum, even though the latter have higher rates of hypertension [28]. It follows that "more health", in terms of total reduction in hypertension, could be realized if the well-to-do population were treated in place of the needier one. But to steer scarce resources away from the poor because their deprivation limits the benefit that they can realize seems to punish them twice over. Existing inequalities in health status would be exacerbated if the resources went to the better off.

Similarly, maximizing strategies face potential conflicts with norms of universality and inclusiveness. Consider a region in which 80 percent of the population lives on the plain and the remainder in inaccessible highland villages. A vaccination campaign with limited funds has just enough money to vaccinate the 80 percent, but given the much higher cost of vaccinating the mountain-dwellers, they would be left out. Suppose that a donor provides the funds necessary to vaccinate the remaining 20 percent. This would achieve inclusiveness, and offer equal treatment. But a maximizing health resource allocator might choose instead to vaccinate the same 80 percent who live in the plain for a second disease if, as is highly likely, the result would be a greater gain in mortality and morbidity.

Allocators must also decide between targeting inequalities and attending to absolute deprivation. Some Latin American countries are among the world's most unequal, but people in the lower social strata in these nations tend to be better off than their counterparts in sub-Saharan Africa [29]. Should the objective be to reduce inequality, or to raise the level of the worst-off as high as possible? In poor countries where meager health budgets are spent largely on a handful of tertiary care hospitals, following a rule of maximization is practically the same strategy as narrowing inequalities. And measures that help the worst-off tend to decrease inequalities.

Ethics and research involving human subjects

During the decades that followed the Second World War, scientists throughout the world came to accept the need for commonly accepted standards of conduct for scientists and prior ethical review of experiments involving human subjects. A trial of German physicians who conducted medical experiments under the Nazi regime was held in Nuremberg, and upon their conviction the court offered a code of conduct that remains the basis for ethical evaluation of research. The World Medical Association, a group created to restore the good name of the medical profession after the horrors of the war years, issued its Declaration of Helsinki in 1964. Revised five times subsequently, the Declaration expanded the scope of the Nuremberg Code and is the most widely cited standard of conduct today. A set of guidelines published in 1993 by the Council of International Organizations of Medical Sciences (CIOMS), a nongovernmental organization established by WHO and UNESCO, has served as an elaboration of the Declaration of Helsinki [30]. The CIOMS guidelines, too, are periodically revised.

These international standards, and the process of prior ethical review to which research is now subjected, have served both scientists and the public well. Although originally resisted by many scientists as a bureaucratic intrusion on their work, these review committees are more often seen as a key element in the social contract under which scientists are authorized to recruit ordinary citizens for their experiments. The public, in turn, is given an assurance that they will not be asked to participate in an experiment unless it has been carefully examined by a group of scientists and laymen, with attention paid both to the frankness of the scientists' disclosure of risks and benefits, and the adoption of any needed protection for the participants.

But not all is well in this field. Even in the richest countries, review committees are overwhelmed by their workload and short of staff, resulting at times in long delays before approving projects. The expansion of the scope of the committee's deliberations, including not only new fields such as population genetics, but also novel aspects of all research, such as conflict of interest, stretches the committees' expertise and adds to expense and delay. Numerous reviews of the system of ethical scrutiny that have been conducted by agencies of the US government have portrayed a system undergoing stress; and the American system is widely regarded as the world's best-developed and certainly its most lavishly funded.

The system of ethical review of research involving human subjects works best for the kinds of studies it was intended to oversee: conventional medical research projects funded and carried out in the same developed country in which the review takes place. The Declaration of Helsinki, created to prevent any recurrence of the Nazi-era abuses, is designed to ensure that no minority will be deprived of the protections given to fellow-citizens enrolled in medical research.

For this very reason, however, the existing system of ethical review, including both the committees and the international guidelines, have faced difficulties in connection with global public health. The latter typically involves sponsors and scientists from a wealthy country working in a poor one, usually in collaboration with nationals of the latter. Following established procedures, collaborative research is to be reviewed at all the institutions of the several participants, and must be approved by all of them. But review committees in many poor countries have been few in number until very recently. Resources, such as staff support and even photo copying, have been hard to come by. Research in epidemiology and other sciences specific to public health presents further challenges, since the issues require expertise that is often lacking. The building of capacity for ethical review in developing countries is a high priority and must be supported and funded by national and international organizations.

The most significant ethical problems in global public health research, however, involve substance rather than process. In international health research involving developing countries, the treatment given to participants in the research is often superior to that available to their fellow-citizens. Nevertheless, a number of international collaborative trials have been subjected to vociferous ethical criticism. In the critics' view, the basic question is whether scientists are using a single standard of ethical conduct [31]. If they are, according to this view, then any experiment they would perform in a poor country must be one that would be permitted in their home countries. The studies that were most strongly criticized did not meet that standard. Whether this is an appropriate standard, however, is another matter entirely. As many observers have pointed out, it would seem to rule out any attempt to gauge the efficacy and safety of a new, inexpensive, affordable treatment if a better therapy were on the market, regardless of its cost (Box 13.2).

Box 13.2 Testing a vaccine

A US-based company developed a vaccine against HIV-1 that appeared promising in animal studies. Phase I trials demonstrated that the vaccine was safe and produced significant antibody levels in most volunteers. The company then wanted to begin phase II trials and decided to carry out the study in Bangkok, Thailand where previous surveillance had identified a cohort of intravenous drug users (IUD) with a high rate of conversion to HIV-1 (of the same strain to which the vaccine had been developed). The company agreed to cover the cost of the study and further agreed to give the vaccine free of charge to the IDU population of the city and at cost to the country for five years, if it proved effective. The study was to be a randomized double-blind prospective study with one group receiving the vaccine and the other tetanus toxoid. All potential participants were to be tested for HIV-1 prior to being enrolled in the study. If they were HIV+ they were referred to one of the municipal hospitals in Bangkok where HIV+ patients were treated by the standard method recommended by the Ministry of Health. This meant that all infections were treated but that control patients were not given antiretroviral therapy. The Municipal Corporation would provide lifetime care. The proposal was reviewed by the Ethical Review Boards of the company and the Thai Ministry of Health and approved. An AIDS activist group strongly objected to the fact that the study did not provide state-of-the-art care for those who became HIV+ during the study. They argued the study would not have been approved in the United States and that the only reason it was being conducted in Thailand was because of the reduced cost. The company countered that the use of state-of-the art therapy would in itself be unethical because the treatment regime would not be sustainable in Thailand and only a small group would have access to this therapy. By offering the best care available in the world, the study would be giving an unfair inducement to the participants. The Ministry of Health agreed with the company.

This study raises several ethical questions. Is the study unethical because participants are not being offered the best care available in the world if they become HIV+? Should the vaccine be tested if it is presently unaffordable to the country? If the developer of the vaccine had been a small local Thai company, would the use of "best available treatment" compared with "standard local therapy" be viewed differently?

There are other areas of controversy in international collaborative public health research. Conflicts of interest among researchers and institutions are a growing problem [32]. Host nations are beginning to insist on some kind of broader community benefit if their citizens are to be used as experimental material. Concern is also growing that methods of informing potential subjects and obtaining their uncoerced, informed, consent are inadequate and insufficiently monitored.

Resources for ethics

The profession of public health lags far behind clinical medicine and biotechnology in focusing attention on ethical issues. While courses in ethics are now standard in medical schools, they have been rare in schools of public health until very recently [33]. Texts are only now beginning to appear [34]. Nevertheless, the trend toward explicit consideration of ethical issues in public health education and institutions is unmistakable. In many countries, the advent of national bioethics commissions and governmental bioethics agencies provides a public forum for deliberation on these issues [35]. The WHO is launching an initiative on ethics and health, following similar actions in several of its regional offices. A global professional society, the International Association of Bioethics, holds world congresses biannually which offer forums for discussion of ethical issues in public health, with particular emphasis on developing countries.

Conclusion

Scholarly consideration of ethical issues in global public health is less well developed than the ethics of clinical medicine. If anything, the ethical issues in global public health are more important, if only because they involve a greater number people who are more vulnerable to exploitation, abuse, and disease. Further efforts to advance deliberations in ethics, both in policy and in scholarship, will benefit those served by workers in global public health.

References

[1] Kass NE. An ethics framework for public health. *Am Public Health* 2001; **91**: 1776–82. A proposed Public Health Code of Ethics, written by a working group of the Public Health Leadership Society, is posted on the website of the American Public Health Association at http://www.apha.org/codeofethics/ (accessed 27 March 2002).

[2] Roberts MJ, Reich MR. Ethical analysis in public health. *Lancet* 2002; **359**: 1055–9.

[3] Thomas A. *Street Price: A Global Approach to Drug Pricing for Developing Countries*. London: VSO, 2001.

[4] Scruton R. WHO, what and why?: Transnational government, legitimacy and the World Health Organization. London: Institute of Economic Affairs; 2000. Also: Scruton R. Tobacco and Freedom. Wall Street Journal (European edition) 2000 January 7.

[5] National Bioethics Advisory Commission (USA). Ethical and Policy Issues in International Research: Clinical Trials in Developing Countries. Bethesda (Maryland): National Bioethics Advisory Commission; 2001.

[6] Warren CW, Riley L, Asma S et al. Tobacco use by youth: a surveillance report from the Global Youth Tobacco Survey project. *Bull WHO* 2000: **78**: 868–76.

[7] Macklin R. *Against Relativism: Cultural Diversity and the Search for Ethical Universals in Medicine*. Oxford: Oxford University Press, 1999.

[8] Physicians for Human Rights (Boston, USA). The problem of dual loyalty: standards of conduct for the health professions (work in progress).

[9] Callahan D, Jennings B. Ethics and public health: forging a strong relationship. *Am J Pub Hth* 2002; **92**: 160–76.

[10] Paul DB. *Controlling Human Heredity: 1865 to the Present*. Atlantic Highlands (New Jersey): Humanities Press, 1995.

[11] Bayer R, Healton C. Controlling AIDS in Cuba. the logic of quarantine. *NEJM* 1989; **320**: 1022–4.

[12] Mann JM. Medicine and public health, ethics, and human rights. *The Hastings Center Report* 1997; **29**: 6–13.

[13] Burr C. The AIDS exception: privacy vs. public health. In: DE Beauchamp, B Steinbock (eds.), *New Ethics for the Public's Health*. Oxford: Oxford University Press, 1999, pp. 211–24.

[14] Wikler D, Beauchamp DE. Lifestyles and public health. In: WT Reich (ed.), *The Encyclopedia of Bioethics*. New York: Simon and Schuster Macmillan, 1995, pp. 1366–9.

[15] Fitzpatrick M. *The Tyranny of Health: Doctors and the Regulation of Lifestyle*. London: Routledge, 2001.

[16] Leichter, HM. *Free to be foolish. Politics and Health Promotion in the United States and Great Britain*. Princeton: Princeton University Press, 1991; Callahan D (ed.) *Promoting Healthy Behavior—How Much Freedom? Whose Responsibility?* Washington DC: Georgetown University Press, 2001.

[17] Eddy DM. The individual vs society: is there a conflict? *JAMA* 1991; **265**: 1446, 1449–50. Also: Eddy DM. The individual vs society: resolving the conflict. *JAMA* 1991; **265**: 2399–401, 2405–6. Also: Emanuel EJ. Patient v. population: resolving the ethical dilemmas posed by treating patients as members of populations. In: M Danis, C Clancy, LR Churchill (eds.), *Ethical*

Dimensions of Health Policy. Oxford: Oxford University Press; 2002, pp. 227–45.

[18] Guindon GE, Tobin S, Yach D. Trends and affordability of cigarette prices: ample room for tax increases and related health gains. *Tobacco Control* 2002; **11**: 35–43. Also: Groosman M, Chaloupka FJ. Cigarette taxes: the straw to break the camel's back. *Public Health Rep* 1997; **112**: 290–7.

[19] UnitedHealth Foundation. America's Health: United Health Foundation State Health Rankings 2001. Edition. Accessed at http://www.unitedhealthfoundation.org/rankings2001/rankings.html, 30 March 2002.

[20] Rose G. *The Strategy of Preventive Medicine* Oxford: Oxford University Press, 1993.

[21] Tucker KL, Mahnken B, Wilson PW et al. Folic acid fortification of the food supply. potential benefits and risks for the elderly population. *JAMA* 1996; **276**: 1879–85.

[22] Breese JS, Glass RI, Ivanoff B, Gentsch JR. Current status and future priorities for rotavirus vaccine development, evaluation, and implementation in developing countries. *Vaccine* 1999; **17**: 2207–22.

[23] World Health Organization. Report of the meeting on future directions for rotavirus vaccine research in developing countries. WHO document *WHO/V&B/00.23.* Geneva: World Health Organization; 2000.

[24] Battin M, Rhodes R, Silvers A. *Justice in Medicine and Health Care.* New York: Oxford University Press, forthcoming; Wikler D, Marchand S. Macroallocation of health care resources. In: P Singer, H Kuhse (eds.), *Companion to Bioethics.* Oxford: Blackwell, 1998. Wikler D, Murray C, *Fairness and Goodness: Ethical Issues In Health Resource Allocation* Geneva: World Health Organization, forthcoming; S Anand, F Peter, A Sen (eds.) *Health, Ethics, and Equity.* Oxford: Oxford University Press, forthcoming.

[25] Menzel P, Marthe Gold et al. Toward a broader view of values in cost-effectiveness analysis of health. *Hastings Center Report* 1999; **29**: 7–15.

[26] Murray C. Rethinking DALYs. In: C Murray, A Lopez (eds.), *The Global Burden of Disease.* WHO/Harvard University Press, 1996.

[27] Nord E. *Cost-Value Analysis in health Care: Making Sense out of QALYs.* Cambridge: Cambridge University Press, 1999.

[28] Stason WB, Weinstein MC. Public-health rounds at the Harvard School of Public Health. Allocation of resources to manage hypertension. *NEJM* 1977; **296**: 732–9.

[29] Gwatkin DR. Health inequalities and the health of the poor: What do we know? What can we do? *Bull WHO* 2000; **78**: 3–18.

[30] Bankowski Z. *International Ethical Guidelines for Biomedical Research Involving Human Subjects.* Geneva: Council for International Organizations of Medical Sciences, 1993.

[31] Angell M. Ethics of clinical research in the third world. *NEJM* 1997; **337**: 847–9; *NEJM* 1988; **319**: 1081–3; Lurie P, Wolfe SE. Unethical trials of

interventions to reduce perinatal transmission of the Human
Immunodeficiency Virus in developing countries. *NEJM* 1997; **337**: 853–6.

[32] Lo B, Wolf LE, Berkeley A. Conflict of interest policies for investigators in
clinical trials. *NEJM* 2000; **343**: 1616–20.

[33] Coughlin SS, Katz VVH, Mattison DR. Ethics instruction at schools of public
health in the United States. *Am J Pub Hlth* 2000; **90**: 768–70.

[34] Beauchamp DE, Steinbock B (eds.). *New Ethics for the Public's Health.*
Oxford: Oxford University Press; 1999; Coughlin SS, Beauchamp TL (eds.),
Ethics and Epidemiology. New York, NY: Oxford University Press, 1998.

[35] Bulger RE, Bobby EM, Fineberg HV (eds.). *Society's Choices: Social and
Ethical Decision Making in Biomedicine.* Washington: National Academy
Press, 1995.

Chapter 14

Putting the public into public health: Towards a more people-centred approach

John Raeburn and Sarah Macfarlane

Introduction

The public health challenges described in this book may generate a sense of disempowerment. Many of the global and national determinants of health seem to be largely out of our control (see Chapter 1). Some people are able to attempt to change the way things are done, but most do not have this opportunity: "We poor people are invisible to others—just as blind people cannot see, they cannot see us." [1]

There have been many public health achievements over the past century. However, the new challenges require a coordinated response from a multiplicity of players (Chapters 1 and 2). The predominantly epidemiological skills of public health practitioners are not sufficient to meet the new challenges. It will be necessary to broaden responsibility for public health beyond a single professional model. We argue that the *public*, as members of communities, or as employees of multi-disciplinary public health organizations, should drive the *public health agenda*; public health practitioners, policy makers and researchers should be trained to partner with communities in the formulation of public health priorities, programmes and values.

The evolution of public health

The term "public health" is used in a variety of ways, for example as a condition, an activity, a discipline, a profession, an infrastructure, a philosophy, or even as a movement (Chapter 1). The term is given attributes and responsibilities, and presented with huge challenges and then judged. Yet, it is not clear where the ownership of public health lies. Common to most of the definitions, usually of public health as a discipline, is a sense of the public interest: "the art and science of preventing disease, promoting health, and prolonging life through the organised efforts of society"; [2] "the committee defines the mission of public health as fulfilling society's interests in assuring conditions in which people can be healthy". [3] But when "public health fails", who exactly fails?, When "public health succeeds", who exactly succeeds? When public health is "at the crossroads", who exactly chooses the direction?

The modern concept of public health originated some two-hundred years ago in Europe and the United States when fear of morbidity and mortality from infectious diseases stimulated scientists, social workers, statisticians, religious leaders, philanthropists and governments to search for ways to protect the public's health. It was quickly understood that disease outbreaks were associated with poverty and poor sanitary conditions and later, as the germ theory matured, medical interventions became significant. In the early twentieth century, just as Flexner led the overhaul of American medical schools, John D Rockefeller supported the establishment of schools of public health around the world. From then on, there has been a debate about the nature of the so-called schism introduced between public health and medicine [4].

Public health processes and achievements have been primarily couched in a scientific language through which health problems are described and assessed and solutions are explored and evaluated. With the aim of preventing death, disease, and disability, populations are studied and interventions determined on the basis of epidemiological evidence, in terms, for example, of "disability adjusted life years". Mass public education campaigns are designed, implemented and evaluated by technical experts. Human issues of suffering and distress and the potential for happiness, health and wellbeing, are summarized in terms such as "risk factors", "social capital", "social determinants" and "equity".

In addition to its scientific requirements and focus on narrowly defined disease conditions, public health can use other epistemologies—such as those of a more qualitative nature—and also investigate issues of quality of life, wellbeing, good health and social justice on a worldwide basis. A significant early expression of this approach was the Declaration of Alma Ata in 1978, in which primary health care was described as "essential health care based on practical, scientifically sound and socially acceptable methods and technology made universally acceptable to individuals and families in the community through their full participation and at a cost that the community and country can afford to maintain at every stage on their development in the spirit of self-reliance and self-determination". [5]

Sadly, the spirit of Alma-Ata was replaced by top-down selective vertical disease-based initiatives that are still being generated today [6].

In 1986 the Ottawa Charter for Health Promotion, subtitled "The New Public Health", redefined the concept of health promotion. The Charter defined health as being "created by caring for oneself and others, by being able to take decisions and have control over one's life circumstances, and by ensuring that the society one lives in creates conditions that allow the attainment of health by all its members". [7] The Charter provided five action streams—a checklist for what needs to be done to promote health at a societal and local level: to build healthy public policy; create supportive environments; strengthen community action; develop personal skills; and reorient health services to a health promotion perspective. The term "health promotion" was added to that of "health protection" as a core activity for public health. Some governments now define public health as health protection plus health promotion [8]. The term "health protection" refers to the more regulatory, centralized and reactive aspect of public health; "health promotion" is more self-determined, community based and developmental. In 1997, the Jakarta Declaration on Health Promotion placed a high priority on promoting social responsibility for health, as well as recognising an important role for the commercial sector in promoting health [9]. The characteristics of "people centered" approaches are contrasted in Table 14.1 with the more conventional epidemiological approach to public health.

In December 2000, about 1500 participants from international organizations and civil society groups came together at the People's Health Assembly in Dhaka, Bangladesh, in order to return the goals of Alma-Ata to the development agenda. A People's Charter for Health was prepared as a call for action to treat health as a human right, tackle the broader determinants of health, develop a people-centered health sector, and ensure people's participation for a healthy world [10].

As individuals and members of communities, we each have responsibility for our own health, for our children's health and for other people's health through commonly accepted or legally enforced behavior. As members of populations, we expect to be protected by our governments and by international agencies. In order to maintain the public's health, international, national and local public health infrastructures have been created and public health professionals are appointed to work for our common good. But there is evidence that this process is not working fairly; for example, the tremendos burden of disease in poor populations and the increasing inequalities between population groups. A commonly promoted solution is for international and national systems to measure and monitor inequalities,

Table 14.1 Contrasting approaches to public health

	Orthodox	People-centered
Groups of interest	Populations, at-risk groups	Aggregations (communities, cultures, etc.)
Aims	Containing and lowering premature death, disease, and disability	Enhancing health, wellbeing and quality of life
Values	Social justice, equity, human rights, social issues, prevention of suffering, science	Empowerment, self-determination, community, culture, diversity, equity, enhancement of quality of life
Means of knowledge building	Epidemiology, evidence-based, rigorous study designs	Participatory, qualitative, quasi experimental, evaluative
Conceptual drivers	Risk, disease, prevention, "medical model," determinants of disease	Health and wellbeing, promotion, people, empowerment, community, "social model," determinants of health
Means of intervention	Policy, population interventions, regulation, media, education and early treatment	Community development, self-determined and participatory action, information and resourcing, action based on community choices
Professional approach	Planning, policy development, expert—driven decisions and priorities, intersectoral collaboration among services	Facilitation of people-driven priorities, partnerships, enabling community control, resource-getting
Overall feel	Scientific, measured	Passionate, intuitive

and to search for solutions. But, until there is better communication between the public and their appointed servants, the public health practitioners, progress in reducing inequalities will be painfully slow.

The pivotal role of community control

The Ottawa Charter championed a people-centered approach to public health when it defined health promotion as "the process of enabling people to increase control over, and to improve, their health" [7]. The *people* dimension implies a bottom-up, grass-roots perspective—the view of the ordinary person in the context of her or his everyday life, culture, and community. This dimension may be contrasted with the traditional academic, political, bureaucratic, or structural dimension, where analyses of determinants and risk are the dominant discourse, and the view is remote from the subjective realities of ordinary people. The *control* aspect is closely allied to the concept of "empowerment", which is the crucial political and psychological dimension for a more people-centered approach to public health. Power and control issues are seen by some as the principal "cause" of the relation between health status and the social gradient [11]—the further down the social scale, the less the power and control one has as a member of society, and the poorer one's health. The Wilkinson hypothesis on inequality and poor health can be accounted for in these terms [12]— that is, the greater the perceived gap by a poor person of what is possible in a society, the greater the sense of disempowerment, and hence the poorer the health and wellbeing.

An example of a community gaining control occurred in Alkali Lake in British Columbia, Canada, where a First Nations community took control to stop their almost universal intergenerational involvement in alcohol abuse, and became a flourishing, economically and culturally strong community [13]. In Cochran Gardens in St Louis, USA, a community resident, Bertha Gilkey, chair of the local tenants' council, led the transformation of the housing project from being an "ugly urban scar filled with broken windows, graffiti, rubbish, frequent shootings [and] angry and fearful people" to a situation in which "Cochran Gardens high-rises are completely renovated. There is a community center, courtyards, tennis courts, playgrounds . . . health clinics, day-care centers, and a vocational training program." Asked about the ingredients for this success, Gilkey said "self-help, dignity, empowerment, responsibility". [14]

The *enabling* dimension is important for defining the nature of the relationship between those holding the power and resources and the general population. If communities are to be enabled to have more control over their health and its determinants then the resources—financial, knowledge, expertise, facilities—need to be made available to them. Given the relative fragility of community processes in the face of other societal pressures, there must also be policy and legislative structures in place to protect community development. This is especially true in the early phases of community development when networks, organizational structures, resources and capacities are being built to enable people to work together effectively.

A classic example of a community development study in Modello and Homestead Gardens in Florida, USA, shows what can be achieved in work facilitated by a professional [15]. These areas were low-income housing projects, with high rates of crime, drug abuse, teenage pregnancy, child abuse, and violence. Processes included relationship building in the community, parenting classes, leadership identification and training, building a strong parent teacher association that went on to organize many community activities, a tenants council, community initiated residential treatment programmes, job training and tutoring programs. Community morale visibly improved in a short time, and within two years, there were major reductions in most social and health negative indicators, including a 60 percent drop in child abuse, 65 percent reduction in drug trafficking, 50 percent reduction in reported parent and child drug abuse, 80 percent reduction in serious delinquency referrals, and a major reduction in teenage pregnancy.

In 1989, Worldwatch did a survey of community development projects from which it was concluded that "grass-roots groups are our best hope for global prosperity and ecology". [16] The groups embrace workplace co-operatives, suburban parents committees, peasant farmer unions, religious groups and neighbourhood action federations. Their work includes building health centres, schools, creating jobs clearing malarial swamps, education, maternal health, training community health workers, creating water supplies, food supplies, saving rainforests and preserving water reservoirs, most of which have direct health impacts. For example, in Lima's Villa El Salvador district, Peruvians have planted a half-million trees; built twenty-six schools, 150 day-care centers, and 300 community kitchens; and trained hundreds of door-to-door health workers. Despite the extreme poverty of the district's inhabitants and a rapidly increasing population, illiteracy has fallen to three percent, one of the lowest rates in Latin America—and infant mortality is 40 percent below the national average. The major ingredients of success have been a vast network of women's groups and the neighborhood association's democratic administrative structure, which extends down to representatives on each block [16].

Evaluation of public health interventions

There is no clearer demonstration of a public health success than the control of an outbreak of cholera, measles or typhoid just as there is no clearer demonstration of failure than the outbreak of cholera, measles or typhoid. Epidemics can result in the downfall of politicians, the resignation of professionals and the death of many people. It is little wonder that public health interventions that can demonstrate reduction in disease incidence are highly sought after.

The conventional procedures for evaluating public health interventions are based on statistical study design and quantifiable outcome measures in intervention and control populations. Results are reported in terms of reduction in disease rates, increase in uptake of services, or changed behaviour between the groups. Success is demonstrated by the existence of a difference in outcome measure between the groups that is statistically significance. It is difficult and usually not desirable to apply such procedures to interventions that emanate from within the community and this is where the debate about evaluation begins.

Advocates of the people-centered approach point out that intervention studies designed from the top-down are not flexible or participatory enough to formulate and implement solutions that are most agreeable to communities and that their evaluations do not necessarily reflect community values of effectiveness. Advocates of the epidemiological approach, on the other hand, point out that evaluations of community-driven interventions are usually so subjective that there is no way of knowing if they can or should ever be brought to scale.

Methods of evaluating community development projects include a variety of quasi-experimental naturalistic designs, demonstration projects with goal-attainment measures set by communities, and participatory action research. There have been some attempts to build systems of evaluation that serve traditional and "new" (people-centered) public health approaches. Health impact assessment, for example, attempts to assess the way in which policies and interventions affect people's health using a mixture of information gathering techniques [17]. In Eastern Nova Scotia, Canada, The People Assessing Their Health (PATH) project has developed community health impact tools tailored to the special needs of individual communities [18].

There is not a lot of formal, evaluated research available in the mainstream academic literature on people-centered approaches, or even on community development programmes as they relate to public health. There are substantial numbers of informal unpublished evaluation reports. Reviews of injury prevention projects indicate that success is often not high for community-based programs where there is little actual community participation, but where there is significant and meaningful community participation, the opposite may be true [19]. A New Zealand quasi-experimental study involving over 4000 people in an urban locality using a multi-cultural approach with a high degree of community and local government involvement, demonstrated significant reductions in child hospitalisation rates, a significantly higher awareness of injury prevention safety messages, higher rates of seat belt use and better fencing of home swimming pools [20].

For many years, Health Canada (a federal department) has funded rural and urban communities across Canada to undertake their own community health projects, often with consultation from regional experts, but under the control of those communities. These projects are selected from a formal application process and have to meet a number of criteria, one of which is that they be evaluated. In this way, these projects meet the requirement of "community control". Many such projects have been evaluated and the results published in government monographs [21].

There are many empowerment studies of mental health primary prevention and promotion projects and the overall impression is that they can be successful [22]. Programmes involving preschool infants, school aged children and high school students seem especially effective [23]. Most involve the "empowerment" of parents, teachers, and the young people themselves, and those that are most successful with teenagers tend to be the peer led. An excellent early overview of such programmes and their effectiveness has been published [24].

The way forward

The debate about evaluation may have less to do with evaluation as with fundamental differences of opinion about the approaches themselves. The Ottawa Charter philosophy continues to inspire people around the world but its principles have never been taken to scale. From a government perspective, the community development model may be threatening since it gives more "democratic" power to people and communities, and allows resources to be controlled at a local level [25]. The follow-up to Alma-Ata went wrong at least in part because politicians and professionals were not prepared to partner with communities in the pursuit of primary health care. Vertical top-down, the so-called evidence-based, programmes were a means of retaining professional and political control and of maintaining accountability for donors. Although they achieved many successes, such programs damaged the wider vision of Alma Ata. The fate of the People's Health Charter will be closely watched.

Much has changed over the last two decades. For example, there is a greater interest in community participation and development partnerships, a better understanding of the need for democracy in networking and in the setting-up of collaborative projects [26]. There is worldwide concern about rising poverty and resulting health inequalities as evidenced by the World Bank study of the perspectives of poor people [1]. Governments have rallied to provide funds in an attempt to alleviate the escalating burden of infectious diseases such as HIV/AIDS, malaria and tuberculosis in poor countries [6]. Ironically, these efforts mirror very closely the Alma-Ata vision and its consequences, i.e., well-articulated global concern about health inequities followed by a massive series of disease-specific responses from developed to developing countries. Already vulnerable health systems must rally their resources to implement these new, mainly curative, interventions. Public health and its workforce are challenged once more.

It is clear from this and other chapters in this book that public health will need to reinvent itself if it is to meet the new challenges of the twenty-first century. There will be much competition for space on the curriculum of training programmes for the new public health leaders as they will need the skills to act and negotiate both globally and locally. Training systems are required that reflect a more people-centered approach to public health. There are an increasing number of programmes providing a training in health promotion, although not all of these are in public health settings, and not all health promotion strongly pursues the people-centered approach. Within mainstream public health, it appears that most training remains within the current public health orthodoxy.

The role of the international community is to provide a mutually supportive environment, and to lessen the pressures and harness the benefits of globalization to ensure the health of marginalized people everywhere [27]. Serious consideration should be given to redefining the contract between the public and its professionals. This will require professional re-orientation towards a more people-centered approach with more public health involvement in multi-sector community development projects. Advocates of the people-centered approach need to initiate a much wider debate about what is involved for public health professional to develop a language of evaluation and a research agenda that reflect the values of all concerned.

References

[1] Narayan D, Patel R, Schafft K, Rademacher A, Koch-Schulte S. *Voices of the Poor: Can Anyone Hear Us?* Oxford: Oxford University Press, 2000.

[2] Acheson D. *Independent Inquiry into Inequalities in Health*. London: HM Stationery Office, 1998.

[3] Institute of Medicine, Committee for the Study of the Future of Public Health. *The Future of Public Health*. Washington, DC: National Academy Press, 1988.

[4] White KL. *Healing the Schism. Epidemiology, Medicine, and the Public's Health*. New York: Springer, 1991.

[5] Primary Health Care. A Joint Report by the Director General of the World Health Organization and the Executive Director of the United Nations Children's Fund. New York: World Health Organization, 1978.

[6] Brugha R, Walt G. A global health fund: a leap of faith? *BMJ* 2001; **323**: 152–4.

[7] WHO. The Ottawa Charter for Health Promotion. Ottawa, Canada: WHO/Canadian Public Health Association/Health Canada, 1986.

[8] NZ Ministry of Health. Preparing the New Zealand Strategic and Action Plan for Public Health: Discussion Document for Consultation. Wellington: Ministry of Health, 2001.

[9] World Health Organization. *The Jakarta Declaration on Leading Health Promotion into the 21st century*. Geneva: WHO, 1997.

[10] People's Charter for Health. PHA Secretariat, Gonoshasthaya Kendra, Savar, Dhaka, 1344, Bangladesh. http://www.pha2000.org.

[11] Steptoe A, Appels, A. *Stress, Personal Control and Health*. Chichester: Wiley, 1989.

[12] Wilkinson R. *Unhealthy Societies. The Afflictions of Inequality*. London: Routledge, 1996.

[13] Health and Welfare Canada. The story of Alkali Lake [Video]. Ottawa: Health and Welfare Canada, 1983.

[14] Boyte H. People power transforms a St Louis housing project. *Utne reader* 1989; **34**: 46–7.

[15] Mills R. Substance abuse, dropout and delinquency prevention: The Modello/Homestead Gardens public housing early intervention project. Coconut Grove, Fla: RC Mills and Associates, 1990.

[16] Durning A. Grass-roots are our best hope for global prosperity and ecology. *Utne reader* 1989; **34**: 34–49.

[17] Report of an Informal WHO Consultative Meeting. Health impact assessment in development policy and planning. Cartagna, Colombia 28 May 2001. Geneva: WHO, 2002.

[18] People Assessing Their Health Project. http://www.path-ways.ns.ca/flash/index.html. Accessed 23 May 2002.

[19] Klassen T, Mackay M, Moher D, Walker A, Jones A. Community-based prevention interventions. *Unintentional Injuries in Childhood* 2000; **10**: 83–93.

[20] Coggan C, Patterson, P Brewin, M, Hooper, R, Robinson, E. Evaluation of the Waitakere Community Injury Prevention Project. *Injury Prevention* 2000; **6**: 130–4.

[21] Health and Welfare Canada. Project abstracts: Health Promotion Contribution Program, 1981–84. Ottawa: Health and Welfare Canada, 1985.

[22] Health Promotion Wales. Mental Health Promotion: Forty Examples of Effective Intervention. Technical Report No. 21. Cardiff: Health Promotion Wales, 1996.

[23] Raeburn J, Sidaway A. Effectiveness of Mental Health Promotion: A Review. Commissioned Report. Auckland: North Health, 1995.

[24] Pransky J. *Prevention: The Critical Need*. Springfield, MO: Burrell Foundation, 1991.

[25] Raeburn J, Rootman I. *People-Centred Health Promotion*. Chichester: Wiley, 1998.

[26] Lasker RD. *Medicine and Public Health: The Power of Collaboration*. New York: The New York Academy of Medicine, 1997.

[27] Macfarlane S, Racelis M, Muli-Musiine F. Public health in developing countries. *Lancet* 2000; **356**: 841–6.

Chapter 15

Strengthening public health for the new era

Robert Beaglehole and Ruth Bonita

This chapter summarizes the state of global public health and suggests the way forward for promoting the practice of public health. We begin by reviewing the main themes from the earlier chapters: the daunting context; the weakness of the public health infrastructure and workforce; the broad scope of public health; and the possibility of a renaissance of public health. We describe our vision for public health and outline the steps required to achieve this vision. We emphasize the need to strengthen both public health training, especially at the postgraduate level, and the ability of public health practitioners to carry out their multiple activities, especially at the country level. Although the focus is on developing countries, strengthening of public health training and practise is required in all countries. Hopefully, we are entering a new era in which the public health perspective will become more central to the health development agenda.

The state of global public health

The daunting global context

The first general theme of earlier chapters is that, despite impressive health gains in almost all countries over the last few decades, the challenges facing public health practitioners remain great—and are often more difficult to address than in the past (Chapters 1 and 2). The unfinished agenda of the control of communicable diseases, for example malaria and tuberculosis, is now compounded by the emergence of new pandemics, notably HIV/AIDS and noncommunicable diseases (NCD), the effects of violence, and global environmental changes.

It is encouraging that some (mostly wealthy) countries have the essentially preventable epidemic of HIV/AIDS more or less under control.

These successes have been achieved at great cost and are primarily due to preventive campaigns, the availability of effective drugs, and to the presence of the appropriate health service infrastructure. However, in many countries in Africa and Asia the HIV/AIDS epidemic is affecting large segments of the population and overwhelming already-stretched health services. A strong economic case can be made for prioritizing the prevention of HIV/AIDS in Africa [1]. Cheap antiretroviral drugs are not yet available for the majority of patients—despite recent reductions in prices and donations—and the health service infrastructure in most countries is not adequate to cope with the escalating case load. Fortunately, some developing countries have demonstrated that good progress in controlling the epidemic is possible, but this requires strong and sustained political leadership together with new resources [2]. The need for strong leadership for public health more generally is one we return to later.

In addition to the continuing communicable disease burden, there is a rapidly growing global burden of NCD and mental health problems (Chapter 2). The burden is largely a consequence of the ageing of populations, due to falling infant and child mortality rates, and lower fertility. Public health programs have contributed to these trends, although many other factors have been important, most notably female education and empowerment [3]. Unfortunately, the information base for estimates of future trends in NCD and mental health problems is still far from complete, despite recent methodological developments (Chapter 2).

In addition, there are newly recognized public health problems such as those related to economic globalization and its impact on wealth creation and distribution, the effects of violence in all its manifestations—especially against women and children [4], global environmental changes and threats to the sustainability of human well-being and health [5]. The globalization of the marketing techniques now being used to such great effect by transnational corporations—such as the tobacco, food, and beverage industries—are contributing to the growing burden of NCD. As discussed in Chapter 1, these challenges present particular problems for public health scientists; the usual study designs are not helpful in assessing the potential future risks to health from, for example, global warming. New methods and new partnerships with scientists in fields outside the health arena are essential for developing credible projections of likely health effects of these global changes. Even when these projections appear robust, it is difficult to ensure the support of policy makers to implement the necessary changes because of the powerful interest groups involved.

The public health implications of global environmental changes illustrate the difficulties facing public health practitioners. Although many environmental scientists are pessimistic about the state of the world and its likely near-term future, others assert that all is well and that general environmental conditions are improving [6]. Unfortunately, the prosperity of industrial economies in recent decades has not created new wealth; it depended on drawing upon ecological "capital." The world has been operating in ecological deficit for decades, extracting resources to the annual value of US$22–30 trillion, without restoring the capital ecological balance [7]. This exploitation of natural resources in the interests of economic growth cannot continue indefinitely.

The prognosis for the future well being of the earth and the health of its human inhabitants is a dire one (Chapter 1). One positive suggestion is for economic investment in wildernesses, especially tropical zone rain forests [8]. There are also economic and health benefits of innovative energy saving and pollution-reducing modifications for large cities [9]. In short, far from the crippling costs to the economy of implementing the Kyoto Accords as predicted by some interest groups, the global economy would experience long-term gains from greenhouse gas reductions and improved population health. The proposals of the Kyoto Accord on global warming highlight the problems faced by public health practitioners when dealing with global issues. The United States, a major contributor to the global problem, has declined to take part in the treaty which addresses the projected impact of global warming, preferring to protect national economic growth, even though this sustained growth will further exacerbate the environmental problem and its public health consequences. The irony is that the economy would experience long-term gains from greenhouse gas reductions as well as improved population health. It remains to be seen whether the need of the United States for support for its global anti-terrorist actions will be sufficient for it to reengage on other pressing global health concerns (Chapter 12). At the time of writing it is hard to be optimistic, given the recent decisions to implement more measures to protect US steel and agricultural interests.

The general issue, and one which extends beyond the domain of public health, is the sustainability of human society; the over-consumption of natural resources by people in wealthy countries severely constrains the ability of poor populations to improve their standard of living (Chapter 1). Given the low likelihood of technical solutions to global environmental issues, the only long-term solution is for wealthy populations to reduce the extravagant nature of their standard of living and the over-consumption of natural resources on which it is based. We need to move towards sustainable global patterns of living, rather than those based on excessive consumption by a minority. The Rio + 10 World Summit on Sustainable

Development held in August, 2002 may stimulate some wealthy countries to develop long term solutions to the complex issues of the environmental effects of economic development.

The public health workforce

The public health workforce contributes to the organization, delivery, and evaluation of health services directed towards both individuals and populations. All countries have a public health workforce of varying organizational patterns [10]. An effective public health workforce is essential for the task of improving health system performance, especially in developing countries. It is also central to the process of building intersectoral activities to ensure that the underlying determinants of population health status are addressed.

The public health workforce is characterized by its diversity and complexity; it includes people from a wide range of occupational backgrounds who are involved in protecting and promoting the collective health of whole or specific populations (as distinct from activities directed to the care of individuals) [11]. In a few countries, notably the United States, it is also involved in ensuring health care for poor populations (Chapter 6).

The second major theme from the earlier chapters is that in all countries and regions described in this book, the public health workforce is not in a position to respond appropriately to the old, let alone the new, challenges (Chapters 7 and 8). With very few exceptions, governments have neglected public health workforce development and the public health infrastructure in general. For too long human resource issues were left to be solved by the market. There needs to be greater attention to planning human resource development and retention, including public health human resources, in the context of a much greater international mobility of the workforce.

In all countries the proportion of the health budget allocated to public health activities is less than 5 percent, and usually of the order of 1–2 percent. This deplorable state of affairs is found in wealthy countries, such as the United States where the public health system had been seriously underfunded for more than thirty years [12], and to an even greater extent in poor countries. Workforce issues are complex and include size, composition, balance between medical and other health science graduates, training methods and skills acquisition, and migration. Secure career pathways and appropriate remuneration packages are of great importance in all countries. In addition, training programs require evaluation and the performance of the workforce requires assessment. Building the public health workforce is a long-term undertaking and will require a substantial commitment of new resources from all countries and donor agencies.

The scope of public health

The third theme is the need to clarify the scope of public health practice. All would agree that public health extends well outside the health sector, yet we are hampered by insufficient experience of effective intersectoral action and a lack of preparation for confronting the new challenges. The development and implementation of comprehensive tobacco control policies in many countries provides one positive example. The World Bank has played an important role in building the evidence base for essential economic policies for effective tobacco control, especially in developing countries [13]. The World Health Organization (WHO) is promoting the Framework Convention on Tobacco Control, the first public health treaty led by the Organization, with ramifications well beyond the health sector [14].

The events of 11 September 2001 in New York, the subsequent "war on terrorism," and the anthrax attacks in the United States have further widened the scope of public health (Chapter 12). The resources provided for the public health response to these events implies that both financial and human resources have been diverted from mainstream public health activities.

The renaissance of public health

The fourth theme from earlier chapters offers some cause for optimism. There are cautious grounds for suggesting that a renaissance of public health is beginning. In Sweden (Chapter 4), and, to a lesser extent in the United Kingdom (Chapter 3) and Australia and New Zealand (Chapter 11), there is political support for public health and an expressed determination to confront health inequalities. Translating this rhetoric into effective programs, however, is much more difficult and serious progress is yet to be achieved. Sweden offers one positive example (Chapter 4).

Fortunately, effective interventions exist against the few diseases which account for most of the excess premature mortality in poor populations [15]. It is increasingly recognized that achieving high coverage of these interventions requires not only new financial resources, but also a well-functioning health system. The public health infrastructure is a key component of health systems. In the effort to support the delivery of vertical disease control programs, this infrastructure has been neglected and marginalized. There are examples of innovative approaches to public health training that may herald the strengthening of the public health workforce in developing countries (Chapters 8 and 10).

From a global perspective, health improvement is increasingly on the development agenda. This new focus on health is in large part due to the efforts of the Director General of WHO; Dr. Brundtland has been an effective advocate for health improvement as a key component of economic and social development in poor countries [16]. This advocacy has contributed to the development of the Global Fund to Fight AIDS, Tuberculosis, and Malaria [17] and the Report of the Commission on Macroeconomics and Health [18] referred to in earlier chapters. It remains to be seen whether this visibility can be maintained and the necessary resources made available for a broad WHO agenda at a time when the United States is taking an increasingly isolationist view of global affairs. This will be a major challenge for the new Director-General of WHO.

A vision for public health

There are at least five interrelated general features which would characterize a reinvigorated practice of public health:

1. Public health practitioners will lead the response to immediate health crises, for example HIV/AIDS, and to emerging problems such as the health impact of global environmental change.

2. Public health practitioners will lead the ongoing health sector reforms which, in turn, will be driven by the need to improve population health rather than by the need to contain costs.

3. Public health practitioners will be promoting intersectoral actions for health improvement and the reduction of health inequalities.

4. Public health research, training and practice will be a high priority in all health services and there will be adequate resources for public health practitioners to tackle a broad agenda. Public health research will clarify the ways diverse policies affect the health of the public. Public health practice will underpin timely and policy relevant information and surveillance systems for both communicable and NCD and will be informed by global and regional perspectives.

5. The values of public health will be explicit and mutually reinforcing interactions will be established between practitioners and the communities they serve.

Achieving this vision

Broadening the scope of public health

A critical step in the reinvigoration of public health practice is for the workforce, in all its diversity, to affirm its professional commitment to a broad view of its mission, including the values of equity and ecological sustainability. A useful beginning to this process would be to include these issues in all public health training programs and shift the focus of public health practice to overall population health improvement. Reducing social and economic deprivation has the potential to reduce the readily preventable burden of disease, both communicable and noncommunicable, especially among disadvantaged groups. Public health scientists and practitioners can contribute to this goal by clarifying the links between social and economic factors and health status, identifying cost-effective approaches to overall health improvement, and by advocating appropriate policies.

The deplorable health conditions of the poorest countries are now receiving increased attention, as are the major health inequalities in wealthy countries [19]. Achieving the goal of halving the number of people living in absolute poverty by the year 2015, the main Millennium Development Goal adopted at the Millennium Summit of the United Nations in September 2000, would do more to reduce health inequalities and improve global health status than any other measure [20]. Unfortunately, this goal is unlikely to be attainable, given the limited international financial commitments to development. The achievement of this and other broad health goals will require major new resources. These, in turn depend on strong global political leadership. The announcement in 2001 by the Secretary General of the United Nations of the Global Fund to Fight AIDS, Tuberculosis, and Malaria, and the beginning of financial commitments to this fund, suggests that at least some wealthy countries are beginning to take seriously the need to improve the health of poor populations. The Fund has now been formally established and disbursed its first allocation of funds in April 2002 [21]. A point of contention is on the balance between support for vertical disease treatment and control programs—mostly based on the purchase of drugs, vaccines and other commodities—and more general support for building health care systems and public health infrastructures [17]. In the face of pressing disease treatment priorities and the desire for short term results, most of the resources have so far been directed towards treatment programs for the three specific diseases for which the Fund was established; there has been a much smaller emphasis on supporting health systems infrastructures and even less on prevention. Although billed as a public/private partnership, the private sector has contributed little to the fund; and many wealthy countries have not yet made any contribution [21].

The Report of the Commission on Macroeconomics and Health, published by WHO in 2001, makes a strong case for improving the health of the poor on economic grounds, as well as, of course, on direct humanitarian grounds [18]. The Commission suggests, for example, that endemic malaria is responsible for at least a 1 percent per year lower growth rate than would be the case in the absence of the disease; these lower growth rates compound and, over time, have a major effect on national wealth creation. The Commission is forthright in its condemnation of the neglect of international health development by wealthy countries. It argues for large new contributions from the international donor community to support low income and a few middle income countries improve the health status of their populations. The United States has made the largest single contribution, US$500 million, but this is only a small fraction of what is being spent on the response to bioterrorism. While the developing countries themselves need to contribute to this endeavor, because of their fragile economies and debt burdens, the bulk of the resources for health improvement will have to come from wealthy countries. The Commission recommended that the WHO and World Bank, with a steering committee of donor and recipient countries, be given the responsibility of co-ordinating and monitoring the resource mobilization process. Implementing the Commission's recommendations requires an initial focus on building the capacity to utilize the extra resources in an appropriate manner. It is difficult to imagine the rapid achievement of the Commission's recommendations given the debates around other global public–private partnerships [16]. Furthermore, the chances of raising the suggested resources are lower in the post-11 September 2001 environment; the renewed focus on national "self-protection" within the United States has shifted huge resources to the response to bioterrorism. It also remains to be seen whether poor countries have the political will to increase their budgetary commitments to health services.

Strengthening the practice of public health

The core public health activities are monitoring population health status and its determinants; prevention and control of disease, injury and disability; health promotion; and protection of the environment [22]. As we have seen from earlier chapters, few of the core public health functions are carried out to a high standard even in wealthy countries. The effect of the increased attention to essential public health functions, especially in North and Latin America (Chapters 6 and 7), is yet to be assessed, especially among disadvantaged populations

The are several reasons for the universal poor performance of public health practice. The recent ideological ascendancy of neo-liberalism has narrowed the focus of public health; responsibility for health is increasingly located at the personal level as national authorities attempt to reduce their costs [23]. However, the determinants of health, and the most powerful means for health improvement, are increasingly located at the global and regional levels [24]. Since most public health work lies outside of the conventional market framework and remains the responsibility of governments, its "public good" nature must be stressed [25]. Fortunately, the concept of global public goods for health is gaining acceptance and this might assist the improvement of public health practice [26].

WHO is promoting the concept of stewardship of the health system whereby governments have a duty to provide overall leadership for the health system in terms of vision, priorities, and regulatory climate, irrespective of whether the funding for the system comes in full or in part from government sources [27].

The lack of response to health inequalities highlights the current lack of leadership provided by most governments. Reducing health inequalities requires action on the underlying structural determinants of social and economic deprivation [28]. This approach is notably absent from the agenda of governments and public health efforts are mostly targeted at the "downstream" effects of exclusion [29]. These programs are acceptable politically but they are not sufficient. Serious intersectoral action is required. Unfortunately, public health practitioners are not skilled in this type of work; it should be taught and researched in all academic public health programs.

Reinvigorating public health teaching and research

Public health training has a long history, primarily in Europe and in North and Latin America [30,31]. The Rockefeller Foundation was instrumental in establishing many of the most prestigious schools of public health in the early decades of the last century [32]. WHO, UNICEF and other international organizations have, more recently, made major contributions to the training of health personnel in developing countries. However, most of this effort has focused on the training of junior health personnel rather than on public health workers with a relevant postgraduate degree [33]. The International Clinical Epidemiology Network (INCLEN), initiated by the Rockefeller Foundation in the mid-1980s, focused over a twenty-year period on providing epidemiological skills for physicians, but failed to address the needs for a modern public health workforce in a resource constrained setting [34].

From a developing country perspective, traditional approaches to public health training, have several limitations [35]:

+ the emphasis on epidemiology and biostatistics and the relative neglect of other public health sciences;

- the isolation from ministries of health, other health providers, local communities, and other relevant scientific disciplines;
- the emphasis on institution-based teaching and the lack of direct field experience;
- the lack of public health practitioners in the field as role models;
- the consideration of public health as a medical speciality; and
- the high cost of the training programs in North America and Europe.

There is a need to reconnect public health education and research with public health practice. All too often academics, divorced from the communities they serve, have concentrated on research issues of questionable relevance to overall population health improvement and the reduction of health inequalities [36]. It is time to move beyond the exquisite refinement of causal associations and the search for new risk factors, for example for cardiovascular disease, and to focus more on understanding why whole populations are at risk of specific disease constellations [37]. There is also a need to support the broad scope of public health teaching and to resist the temptation to allow molecular epidemiology, clinical epidemiology, and health services management to dominate training and research programs. An innovative project began in 1992 with the launch of the Public Health Schools Without Walls (PHSWOW) initiative in Africa, later expanding to Asia. The program was driven by the energy and initiative of the Rockefeller Foundation; CDC field-based training experience in epidemiology was also of conceptual importance to the new program [38,39]. The guiding principle of the initiative was that public health training should be provided through a combination of rigorous academic and supervised practical experience, with a focus on the capacity to pursue rather than memorise knowledge [35].

The PHSWOW program, and others like it (Chapter 10), aim to train graduates competent to respond to practical health problems and to manage health services, especially at the district level. To achieve this goal, the Ministry of Health plays a significant role in these programs. A feature of the PHSWOW curricula is the substantial period of supervized field training, up to 75 percent of the course. During this time trainees are expected to acquire and demonstrate competence in key areas, including the ability to: investigate important local health problems; design, manage and evaluate health programs; assess and control environmental hazards; and communicate effectively with colleagues, individuals, communities, and policy makers.

A recent evaluation of the program concluded that, despite the lack of clear initial goals and milestones for evaluation, the PHSWOW achievements could provide one foundation on which to build public health capacity in developing countries [40]. There is an opportunity to capitalize on existing public health training programs in developing countries by supporting: their financial stability; faculty development including faculty research capability; development of broad curricula; and the development of secure career paths. Sustained commitment of resources and effort is required to expand the new approach to regional training centres. Given the long-term neglect of planning for the public health workforce—and the rest of the health workforce—in developing countries, a consortium of donors and agencies with a long-term commitment to this goal is required. The WHO is well placed to play a leadership role in this endeavor.

Public health leadership

To capitalize on the potential for the reinvigoration of public health practice, strong political and professional leadership is essential. At the international level there is cause for optimism. The WHO is focusing on a select group of priority issues and on the need to support health improvement for economic reasons. The Commission on Macroeconomics and Health has firmly placed health at the center of the international development agenda. The World Bank, the most important lender for population health improvement, is now taking the underlying determinants of health into consideration in its lending programs [41]. This strengthening of global leadership may also lead to stronger leadership of public health practice at the regional, national and local levels. An educational focus on public health leadership in developing countries is also required to ensure the development of the next generation of leaders who will place public health firmly on their country's agenda.

Modern electronic communication technology can build and support leadership and networks; creative technical and financial innovations are required to overcome the "digital divide," especially in sub-Saharan Africa and South Asia [42]. Training centers in developed countries could contribute to distance learning programs based on the full range of modern technology to support the goals of the training programs in developing countries.

In many countries, academic public health specialists still have the independence and autonomy to play a major public health leadership role. Closer ties between academic public health researchers and public health practitioners at the national level will also increase the value of research. The credibility of public health professionals will be strengthened by closer partnerships with communities, their representatives and other agencies working at the local level [43]. Full community participation in public health activities is the key to more responsive and effective programs (Chapter 14). However, moving from the traditional top down approach to health improvement strategies to a more inclusive model will be difficult for most public health practitioners and this emphasises the importance of a new approach to public health educational programs.

Responding to globalization

Public health practitioners can no longer ignore the impact of globalization on the determinants of population health status at the national level. The key issue is the impact of the liberalization of trade rules on poverty, especially in developing countries. Increasing the developing world's share of global trade would do more to lift people out of poverty than increased aid spending. Can the World Trade Organization (WTO) Multilateral Trade Agreements be interpreted in a way that shifts the balance from protecting the economies of wealthy countries to promoting development where it is most needed [44,45]? Can the huge European Union and US subsidies for agriculture be dismantled in favor of easier access for products from developing countries, without imposing new conditions [46]? These issues have major health implications for poor countries but are only now getting on to the public health agenda.

Comprehensive research and action agendas are required on the globalization and health interface. For example, what are the public health implications of the WTO Multilateral Trade Agreements [47]? What are the health impacts of the global marketing of energy-dense food products, and alcohol and tobacco? What will be the health effects of global environmental changes? The tools available for understanding the process and effects of globalization on population health status are still rudimentary, though environmental health scientists are leading the way. This research agenda provides an exciting opportunity for public health practitioners to take the initiative and position themselves at the forefront of civil society's response to globalization. Until now, the response has been lead by civil society groups who have, for example, made progress by increasing access to affordable drugs which are constrained by the WTO agreement on intellectual property rights (TRIPS). The response from the pubic health community to most globalization and health issues has been, at best, muted [16].

The challenge for the international public health research community is to establish a mechanism for facilitating research that extends beyond national boundaries perhaps through a new style of co-operative research—the public health equivalent of the human genome project. The WHO is in an ideal position to lead this collaborative research agenda.

The WHO could usefully establish a globalization and health research database and associated web site that would include relevant data sets from a range of disciplines and a registry of ongoing and completed research projects. An important research question, and one that the WHO is uniquely qualified to address, is the need to use more comprehensive surveillance data for the full range of diseases at a regional level and to collect new data unconstrained by national boundaries. The research endeavor, as with any another public health problem, is only the first step; hand in hand must go the appropriate public health response. The incorporation of the results of this research into education and learning programs will ensure that the next generation of public health professionals is better equipped to address these emerging global issues.

Both scientists and policy-makers face unfamiliar and difficult challenges in addressing these broad public health issues. It is important to continue to identify, quantify and reduce the risks to health that result from specific, often localised, social, behavioral and environmental factors. It is also important to be increasingly alert to the influences on population health that arise from today's larger-scale social and economic processes and global environmental disturbances. Research within this framework will enhance the capacity to manage social and natural environments in ways that support and sustain population health.

Conclusion

The ultimate goal for public health practitioners is to ensure that the public health perspective is integrated into all health, social and economic policies and programs. Ideally, all public policy should have an explicit commitment to overall health improvement, the reduction of health inequalities, and the sustainability of human societies. These goals are a long way from being realized, in part because this vision is not shared and the public health workforce is not yet equipped for these tasks.

As earlier chapters have emphasised, the challenges facing public health practitioners are huge. However, a reasonably optimistic future for public health can be predicted; several innovative public health training activities are underway; health is now high up the international development agenda; and new funds for health improvement are becoming available. The vision for public health outlined in this book is both necessary and achievable. It is to be hoped that as the reinvigoration of public health practice gathers pace, the public health perspective will become more central to the development process.

References

[1] Creese A, Floyd K, Alban A, Guiness L. Cost-effectiveness of HIV/AIDS interventions in Africa: A systematic review of the evidence. *Lancet* 2002; **359**: 1635–42.

[2] Lamptey PR. Regular review: Reducing heterosexual transmission of HIV in poor countries. *BMJ* 2002; **324**: 207–11.

[3] Caldwell JC. Routes to low mortality in poor countries. *Pop Dev Review* 1986; **12**: 171–220.

[4] Venis S, Horton R. Violence against women: A global burden. *Lancet* 2002; **39**: 1172.

[5] McMichael AJ. Population, environment, disease, and survival: Past patterns, uncertain futures. *Lancet* 2002; **359**: 1145–8.

[6] Lomborg B. *The Sceptical Environmentalist*. Cambridge: Cambridge University Press, 2001.

[7] Costanza R, d'Arge R, de Groot R et al. The value of the world's ecosystem services and natural capital. *Nature* 1997; **387**: 253–60.

[8] Wilson EO. *The Future of Life*. New York: Knopf, 2002.

[9] Suzuki D, Dressel H. *Good News for a Change*. Toronto: Stoddart, 2002.

[10] Porter D. (ed.). *The History of Public Health and the Modern State*. Amsterdam: Editions Rodopi BV, 1994.

[11] Rotem A et al. The Public Health Workforce Education and Training Study: Overview of findings. Canberra: Australian Government Publishing Service, 1995.

[12] McLellan F. CDC chief Koplan quits "the best job in public health". *Lancet* 2002; **359**: 773.

[13] The World Bank. *Curbing the Epidemic*. Washington, DC: The World Bank, 2000.

[14] Yach D, Bettcher D. Globalisation of tobacco industry influence and new global responses. *Tob Control* 2000; **9**: 206–16.

[15] Jha P, Mills A, Hanson K et al. Improving health outcomes of the global poor. *Science* 2002.

[16] Horton R. WHO: the casualties and compromises of renewal. *Lancet* 2002; **359**: 1605–11.

[17] Brugha R, Walt G. A global health fund: A leap of faith? *BMJ* 2001; **323**: 152–4.

[18] Report of the Commission on Macroeconomics and Health. *Macroeconomics and Health: Investing in Health for Development*. Geneva: World Health Organization, 2001.

[19] Independent Inquiry into Inequalities in Health. London: Stationery Office, 1998.

[20] World Health Organization. *World Health Report, 1999*. Geneva: WHO, 1999.

[21] Ramsay S. Global Fund makes historic first round of payments. *Lancet* 2002; **359**: 1581–2.

[22] Bettcher DW, Sapirie SA, Goon EHT. Essential public health functions. *Wld Hlth Stat Quart* 1998; **51**: 44–54.

[23] Beaglehole R, Bonita R. *Public Health at the Crossroads: Achievements and Prospects.* Cambridge: Cambridge University Press, 1997.

[24] Jamison DT, Frenk J, Knaul F. International collective action in health: objectives, functions, and rationale. *Lancet* 1998; **351**: 514–17.

[25] Chen LC, Evans TG, Cash RA. Health as a global public good. In: I Kaul, I Grunberg, MA Stern (eds.). *Global Public Goods.* New York: Oxford University Press, 1999.

[26] Smith R, Beaglehole R, Drager N (eds.). *Global Public Goods for Health.* Oxford: Oxford University Press (in press).

[27] World Health Organization. *World Health Report, 2000.* Geneva: WHO, 2000.

[28] Gepkins A, Gunning-Schepers LJ. Interventions to reduce socio-economic health differences. *Eur J Pub Hlth* 1996; **6**: 218–26.

[29] McKinlay JB, Marceau LD. A tale of three tails. *Am J Public Health* 1999; **89**: 295–8.

[30] Fee E, Acheson R (eds.). *A History of Education in Public Health: Health that Mocks the Doctors' Rules.* Oxford: Oxford University Press, 1991.

[31] Pan American Health Organization. Development of Public Health Education: Challenges for the XXI Century. XIX Conference of the Latin American and Caribbean Association of Public Health Education (ALAESP). Havana, 2–4 July 2000.

[32] Brown ER. *Rockefeller Medicine Men.* Berkeley: University of California Press, 1980.

[33] World Health Organization Technical Report Series No. 717. (1985). Health manpower requirements for the achievement of Health for All by year 2000. WHO Technical Report Series No. 738. (1986). Regulatory mechanisms for nursing training and practice meeting primary health needs. World Health Organization Technical Report Series No. 780 (1989). Strengthening the performance of community health workers in primary health care. World Health Organization Technical Report Series No. 783 (1989). Management of human resources for health.

[34] White KL. *Healing the Schism. Epidemiology, Medicine, and the Public's Health.* New York: Springer, 1991.

[35] Bertrand WE. Public Health Schools Without Walls: New directions for public health resourcing. New York; The Rockefeller Foundation, Draft, March 1999.

[36] Pearce N. Traditional epidemiology, modern epidemiology, and public health. *Am J Pub Hlth* 1996; **86**: 678–83.

[37] Beaglehole R, Magnus P. The search for new risk factors for coronary heart disease: Occupational therapy for epidemiologists. *Int J Epidemiol* 2002 (in press).

[38] Music SI, Schultz MG. Field Epidemiology Training Programs: New international health resources. *JAMA* 1990; **263**: 3309–11.

[39] Goodman RA, Buchler JW, Koplan JP. The epidemiological field investigation. Science and judgement in public health practice. *American J Epidemiology* 1990; **132**: 9–16.

[40] A Report to the Rockefeller Foundation. *Enhancing Public Health in Developing Countries, July 2001.* New York: Rockefeller Foundation, 2001.

[41] Wolfensohn JD. The Other Crisis. Address to the Board of Governors, Washington, D.C. October 6, 1998.

[42] Chandrasekhar CP, Ghosh J. Information and communication technologies and health in low income countries: the potential and the constraints. *Bull WHO* 2001; **79**: 850–5.

[43] Raeburn J, Rootman I. *People-Centred Health Promotion.* Chichester: Wiley, 1997.

[44] Editorial. How to make global trade diminish poverty. *Lancet* 2002; **359**: 1359.

[45] Pollock AM, Price D. Market forces in public health. *Lancet* 2002; **359**: 1363–4.

[46] Lang T, Lobstein T, Robertson A, Baumhofer E. Building a healthy CAP. *Eurohealth* 2001; **7**: 34–40.

[47] Ransom K, Beaglehole R, Correa C et al. The public health implications of the multilateral trade agreements. In: K Lee et al. (eds.). *Health policy in a Globalising World.* Cambridge: Cambridge University Press, 2002.

Index